UNDERSTANDING
YOUR LIFE

UNDERSTANDING YOUR LIFE

A Patient's Guide to Chinese Medicine

Warwick Poon
Dip.Ac., FAACMA, Dip.OM., M.Ac.

©2012

Forres, Scotland

Dedication

This book is dedicated to the women in my family who have taught me more about "Life" than any Traditional Chinese Medicine course ever could. My mother Nellie, my wife Áine, and my two splendid daughters Tabor and Thérèse.

Contents

Part One
Childhood

Part Two
Adulthood

Foreword

Understanding Your Life is a guided tour of life from conception to death. Your guide is Warwick Poon, a gentle, compassionate, humble man who shares his wisdom about life through the lens of Traditional Chinese Medicine. Drawing on his own wealth of experience as a practitioner of Traditional Chinese Medicine, the author explains the perspectives of this ancient tradition on subjects as diverse as self-discipline, relationships, human growth and development, parenting and sex. Originally written as a series of essays this book is drawn together with a narrative thread of life from "How to make the best baby you can" to "Death". The reader can choose to select a chapter of interest or can read from cover to cover.

Understanding Your Life is an intensely personal book with a disarming frankness and honesty. The author shares from his heart some very practical lifestyle advice without any agenda or gestures towards political correctness. This lifestyle advice is always underpinned by explanations drawn from ancient Chinese medical and cultural traditions to help the reader to understand the rationale behind the advice.

Understanding Your Life has something for everyone because it is fundamentally all about our shared experience of being human from cradle to grave.

John McDonald, M.Ac., FAACMA,

Adjunct-Senior Lecturer & PhD candidate,

Microbiology and Immunology Research Group,

School of Medicine,

Griffith University,

Queensland, Australia

Introduction from the Author

The genesis of this project began after spending many hours discussing periods with mothers and daughters in clinic. It became apparent that the mystery of periods was simply that, a mystery. I found that an alternative view of periods was helpful to both mother (who did not know what a good and healthy period was) and daughter (who was about to embark on a lifetime of periods). It became apparent that a short essay would be useful and I wrote this in 1991. With the help of a photocopier I began to distribute these to my patients with great success. As time went on, they began to offer money for the copies when I had run out.

Thanks largely to the efforts of my business partner Tracy and the urging of my patients, I became inspired to compose further essays on subjects that were needed in clinic. Eventually, my wonderful wife suggested I put all the essays together and form them into a book. It has taken over eight years to compile and I have arranged these essays into something that I believe is both useful and makes some kind of sense.

I hope that you find this book enjoyable and I wish you good health.

Warwick Poon

Melbourne, April 2012.

How to Use this Book

This book can be read as a whole, or each short chapter can be read in isolation. I have pitched the book to appeal and be understandable to an early adolescent and hope that it may have some influence for good in young lives, as well as being useful to people of all ages, even if some people find it unsophisticated.

This book is a simplification and compilation of many detailed and complicated theories and is intended only for lay people. It may allow them to understand life from an alternative point of view. The intention is not to suggest that Westerners adopt a traditional viewpoint, but that, in some cases, it is useful to see things differently. Almost no one in the world today comes from a culture that follows the ancient Chinese, but it may be that our current cultural ideas do not always apply well to all situations. I think that it is like driving a car that does not have reverse gear. You don't use it much, but it is useful on occasions.

Scholars and practitioners of Chinese medicine will certainly find some inaccuracies, due to the necessity of simplification, however I do believe that it follows the ideas and concepts of Chinese medicine reasonably well and maintains an overall integrity and internal consistency.

UNDERSTANDING YOUR LIFE

A Patient's Guide to Chinese Medicine

Part One

Childhood

CHAPTER ONE

How to Make the Best Baby You Can

The human body is a complex piece of equipment. There are aspects that can be seen, such as skin, flesh, blood and hair, just as there are aspects that cannot be seen, like emotions, the soul and what the Chinese call Qi (pronounced "chi"). It is fairly easy to understand, at least superficially, how the physical body works. Food is eaten and is broken down into amino acid building blocks and then reconstructed into useful proteins. But what is it that actually makes you, you?

If you are your body, then it should follow that when a leg or arm is cut off, you become less of a person. This is not the case however. If you are the sum of the neurone connections in the brain, then when parts of the brain cease to function, it should follow that parts of you cease to exist, which is also not true.

How about viewing yourself as a small piece of heaven, that is clearly distinct from all other pieces, which requires you to learn some deep and meaningful lessons? With forethought and planning, you descend into the physical world by entering a fertilised egg. As the physical body of the baby is growing, you reside in the centre of the chest (where you find the pumping muscle) and use the brain to control some of the functions of the body. But how is this control achieved? The body is physical, controlled by chemical-electrical impulses, and you are spiritual, with no ability to exert influence in the physical realm.

You require a substance that is not spiritual, and not physical. For the sake of this book, let us call this Qi. This Qi must be almost physical in nature, so that it can exert an impact upon the physical body. It must also be similarly able to affect the emotional and mental realms of the person, so that the spirit can exert its controlling effects on the Qi. It has similarities to magnetism and electricity, but is not the same. If Qi is the link between you and your body, then there must be a way of controlling it, measuring it and even manipulating it.

This is the realm of the Traditional Chinese Medicine practitioner. For at least three thousand years, and some would say several thousand before that, the Chinese have been investigating and codifying this system of medicine. Modern Western thought is beginning to come to the realisation that if the mind is in a certain attitude, then it can cause or heal disease. The modern theories of psycho-immunology are some of the best examples of the new thoughts and realisations within Western thinking.

How can your mind control wellbeing? This occurs through the action of Qi, controlled by the mind. However it is a double-edged sword. The external physical energy will have a particular pattern, which will impact upon a person's Qi pattern and influence the way that person thinks and relates to the world. So individuals from a common geographically located point (town, city, country), with a common upbringing and common problems, will have personality traits in common. They will not be the same as each other, as everyone is born with a different soul, needs to learn different lessons, and is brought up differently, but some traits will definitely be the same or similar.

If the external environment can impact the energy field, and therefore the Qi pattern, so can a person's physical structure. The physical body is closely linked to the Qi pattern. When out of balance it will cause the Qi pattern to become unbalanced too. If the Qi pattern is forced to be out of balance by the physical body, then the Qi will impact on the mental processes and influence the way that that person thinks and feels.

Can physical ailments therefore be diagnosed and treated by non-physical means? The answer is obviously yes. For example, if the Qi feeding the Heart is too hot then you (that is the real, spiritual you) cannot take a holiday from this physical world, which is necessary each night. The Heart is the house where the spirit resides and operates the body's functions. If the Heart is too hot then it becomes a jail and you cannot leave, which you must do in order to sleep, so insomnia results. In mild cases, a lot of dreams are recalled. In severe cases, when the spirit fights to leave, palpitations occur.

Some people allow themselves to get angry at things that normally would not make them angry. This will cause hot Qi to go through their Liver. If they do not control their anger, their eyes become dry and scratchy, they tear tendons and muscles, as well as lose weight. If they are in the right age bracket, they may even suffer a heart attack. In severe cases, they may find that their Liver Qi makes them violent. If not controlled, they will end up incoherent and the men in white suits may very well take them for a holiday in a padded cell.

This is an illustration of how an emotion can cause a physical response, which can then cause hot Qi, causing an emotional response.

When you make babies you use Qi and physical means. The female egg must be physically fertilised by the male, but also a lot of Qi is required for the process to work. Which particular sperm fertilises the egg, and whether or not it fertilises the egg is not random, but dictated by the type of Qi in the parents' energy fields.

Conception is determined somewhat by genetics, but a lot of physical, emotional and personality traits are determined by the Qi that is provided by both parents. In fact, the Qi is condensed, and in this compact form is called Jing. The amount of Jing supplied during the procreative act will determine the strength and potential of the baby's Qi.

Male Jing when combined with the female Jing initiates combat. The male and female Jing fight and produce combinations of male and female in every cell and fibre of the body. Each organ will have a different amount of maleness or femaleness and this will depend on the different and relative strengths of the Jing produced by each parent. The male Jing, if strong will produce a girl, if weaker, a boy. An interesting trend was found among English Navy divers. It seems that all of the divers who work underwater seem to produce daughters. Because diving is under pressure, and the aqualung delivers air at a higher pressure, the divers tend to be healthier. This produces daughters and confirms the Traditional Chinese Medicine (TCM) theory.

The pattern of Qi in each parent at the time of conception produces a chain of events that cannot be stopped or redirected for at least 2-3 years. The personality and health of the person you are creating is dictated by the Qi patterns of the parents at the time of conception. It is for this reason that an understanding of relationships is so important. Whilst this is discussed later, (see Chapter 23) a small understanding is needed here. If your energy pattern is strong in some points and weak in others, then meeting or being with a person from the opposite sex who makes you feel good will probably mean that their strengths will be balancing your weak points. Similarly, their weak points will be balancing your strengths. Because you are both balanced out, you will make a balanced baby, but if you are with someone that makes you more unbalanced, angry and confused or takes your confidence away, then you will make a poor quality baby.

CHAPTER TWO

Jing Qi

If you will accept that Qi is required for the maintenance of all life, then you may ask, "What is its origin?" Traditional Chinese Medicine believes that it is stored in the Kidneys as Jing. Jing is not Qi. Jing is a form of condensed Qi, which can be converted into Qi when required. Jing can be seen as a type of compressed air like that used by a scuba diver. The diver has a mechanical regulator, which supplies the correct amount of air required by the diver for whatever particular depth the diver is diving at. If the compressed air is released without the regulator, then it is lost, unusable, and potentially dangerous.

To continue the analogy, the more air that is released, the deeper the diver may go and the quicker the compressed air is spent. In people, the greater the stresses and damage to the body, the more Jing is required to be released. The mechanical regulator is likened to the function of the Kidneys. Sometimes, but not often, the Kidneys lose their ability to regulate. Too much Jing is released into the body and madness develops, whereas sometimes there is too little Jing and the person develops debilitating diseases, such as chronic fatigue.

It is for this reason that some forms of Qi Gong, yogic and meditation practices should be avoided without proper instruction. If the unwary practice incorrectly or too often, then they open the gate to their Jing. They may feel marvellous and may accomplish miraculous feats but can become out of control and destroy themselves.

There are in China at the moment Qi Gong junkies, who do not eat or sleep and survive entirely on Qi Gong. These people seem to have altered mental states and die very quickly. In India there is a similar medical problem called "Kundalini Syndrome". (The Indian idea of joining the chakras is better known in the West than Chinese theory). This is brought about by raising the Kundalini without due control, the result being the same as the uncontrolled and rapid loss of Jing; an early death and often mania.

There are many legends about martial artists who perform miraculous feats of magic and physical excess. Even at the present time, there are people who can achieve such things. These people call upon their Jing Qi. If they perform these feats too often, they will find themselves with some of the symptoms of Jing deficiency.

Jing should be nurtured and regulated and not wasted. It should only be used when required. Almost everything we do costs us Jing. Sooner or later, it will be depleted, and we will grow old and die. The Oriental mind sees this as a fact of life, which should be delayed for as long as possible. The young respect old people, as they have been able to live longer. It has been said that life is an obstacle course. Do not be ashamed of completing a longer and tougher course than others. So how do we accomplish this?

If an individual undertakes no physical exercise, then the body becomes less serviceable, and sicknesses and stagnations occur. Jing will be utilised to correct and heal these quickly. On the other hand, if a person becomes obsessed with exercises and trains too often then they use Jing at an even more rapid rate. Moderation is the key.

How much is too much or too little is a question only the reader can answer (but first be informed).

Another method of conserving Jing is through our eating habits. Some people modify their diets to include only what they consider "good food". Usually the result is such that the individual does not obtain all the components that their diet requires. Jing is then used as a replacement or supplement, a supplement that theoretically can be used up and never replaced. Other people will rely on "junk food" and Jing will be required to remove the poisons to ensure that they do not create any diseases. Jing should not be used as a protection against bad habits. The only sensible way to approach diet is to make an informed decision, you will then be able to place diet in the correct perspective so that you will not be constantly focusing on it. One of the worst things that a person can do is to become obsessed with what they eat.

From a TCM health practitioner's point of view, Jing is to be used minimally. The practitioner will attempt to conserve Jing and treat a person's ailment by using minimal amounts of Jing.

There is a school of thought in Chinese medicine that encourages the practitioner to use as few needles as possible to get the job done, and points that are as mild as possible. If the concept of Jing is not understood, then it cannot be considered a factor in the selection of treatment. Would you, as a patient prefer to suffer a disease for 3 weeks, instead of one week and a loss of 5-6 years of your life? Ethically, a qualified TCM practitioner will consider the best course of treatment according to his point of view.

The longer you are sick, the more Jing you will use. If the treatment is radical, and causes new problems, (which were not there initially), then Jing is used, not only in the process of the treatment, but also to rectify the damage that has been caused. This may take months, and therefore the total sum of Jing used is far in excess of what is required by a more gentle form of treatment.

Children have a large amount of Jing. You may notice that they heal quickly. They are full of life and problems do not perplex them for long. Even trauma and skin damage, provided it is not too severe, usually heals without scarring. As you progress through life, this ability will decrease. You will know your Jing is becoming low when you cannot call on it as readily, when your hair becomes thin or grey and you develop an overemphasised capacity for fear.

CHAPTER THREE

Earlobes

In the womb, the Jing from parents builds the baby's body, right down to the minute detail. The last parts of the body to be formed are the earlobes. If there is insufficient Jing then the earlobes will be small, or missing. If there is a lot of Jing left over, then the earlobes will be large, thick and contain a lot of flesh.

When the baby is born, the earlobes are one of the first indications of the potential health, personality and length of life of the new person's body. When the earlobes are large, any sicknesses or injuries will be easily overcome. Those without earlobes will require a lot of assistance and will heal poorly. The psychological scars imposed by a poor upbringing will cut more deeply into those without earlobes. As adults, they will be quick to develop and use defence mechanisms. These defence mechanisms will be diverse and well used.

When examining an ear, you can feel the cartilage which produces the hard feeling and much of its shape, and on the outside a thin film of skin which covers the ear. At the base of the ear some flesh is left to sag below the cartilage, like melted wax from a candle. This is the earlobe. Its size and shape give an indication of the potential (and only the potential) of the individual. Some earlobes are close to the head and may even attach. These are the yin type constitutions of inherited Jing. Others grow further from the head. These are the yang type constitutions of inherited Jing.

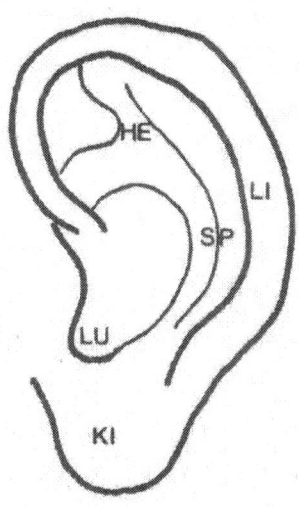

Those with yin type earlobes (growing close to the head) have a lot of inner strength, sleep well, usually develop a double chin, have plenty of flesh on their body, and are not naturally gifted at sport, but can, on occasion show surprising ability. Those with the yang type of earlobe (growing further from the head) are very hot and suffer from hot and feverish diseases, insomnia, do a lot of exercise, are usually thin, and are regularly subject to a loss of temper.

Those who have large, flat-bottomed earlobes, with plenty of flesh on the inside, as well as on the outside are the luckiest. They can do anything, but usually do not, through lack of enthusiasm. Everything comes too easily for them and it requires a lot of intelligence and effort for their parents to bring them up with enough forethought and stimulation so that they can "change the world". If everything seems to come easily to them, then make everything harder for them. Remember, "hard for them now, easy for them later".

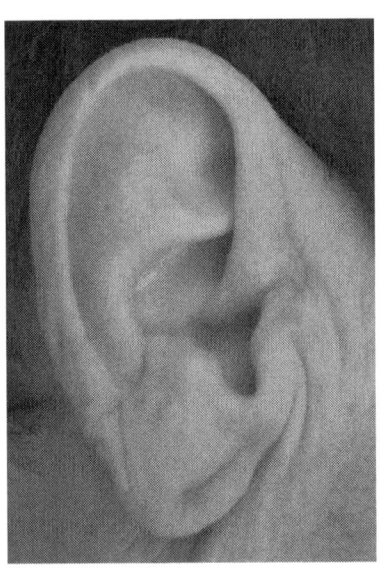

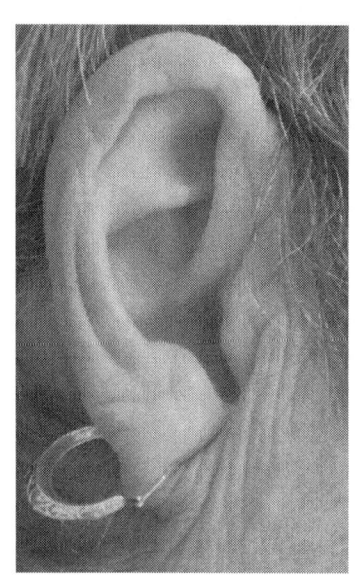

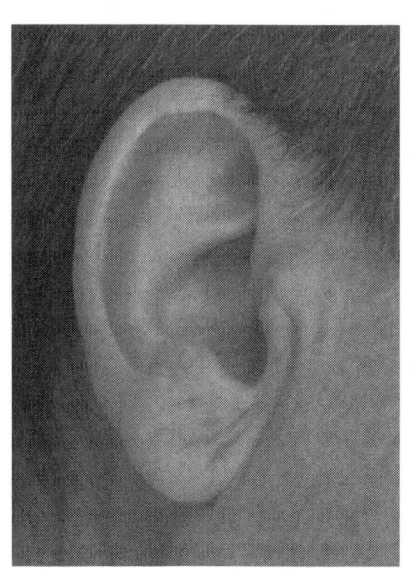

CHAPTER FOUR

Growth & Development

The growth of a baby depends on all Qi functions, but mainly the Ren Mai channel (see below) and Kidney yin. Assuming that the Kidney yin and yang functions are equal and adequate, which is almost impossible; then Kidney yin is called on to produce fluids, blood and flesh. Kidney yang is only required to supply some digestive energy. The rest of its yang energy is used for activating the Lungs and muscles. What do we see in a baby? Abundant yang energy and a distinct lack of ability to sleep. What we would call insomnia in an adult. Yet a baby sleeps many hours to replenish the yin which is being used up. This is a relative excess of yang. Some may even say a true excess of Kidney yang. Where is the yin?

All yin originates in the Kidney yin. Kidney yin is busy building blood, flesh and bone. Its whole effort is concentrated on building a body. Therefore, the usual functions associated with yin are seen as depleted. One of the jobs of Kidney yin is to produce Wei Qi. Little Wei Qi (protective energy) is available, so diseases are easily caught. Any fevers seem to be excessive with no yin cooling. The relatively excessive yang can produce an uprising of Stomach Qi and the baby will vomit easily.

Kidney yin supplies the Qi for nourishing and repair, and the growth of the body. The Ren Mai channel is the passageway through which this Qi ascends to the head.

In the womb, when baby is bent in a circle as a foetus, the Ren Mai has a small role to play. When baby is born, and stretches out, Ren Mai has the major function of allowing the yin Qi to ascend to the head so growth and development will take place. If Kidney yin or the Ren Mai are damaged, either at birth, or prenatally, or even at conception, then delayed or insufficient development will occur.

The Heart organ is the organ that controls intelligence and thoughts. It has control over the voice, in that it controls the tongue, and what is said. The Lung supplies the volume, and we can gauge the relative energy of the Lungs by the volume of the voice. It is only when a baby's heart begins to solidify and become more capable that baby begins to try to talk, not just cry. It is at this time also that intelligence and reason come into play. However, the Heart does not solidify and become strong for a long time. Hence, you cannot use reason and logic when dealing with young children. The Heart is not thinking clearly until around the age of 14-16 years. However, Heart is still King (refer to Chapter 7) and it decides what will happen in the body. Heart, if you like, is the control or discipline of the mind and body.

During childhood, the Heart learns what behaviour is acceptable for it to be healthy, and what it perceives as being unhealthy. When the Heart is well fed and strong, joy and happiness are experienced.

A child's Heart needs to learn how to discipline the other organs, in the same way, as a child needs discipline from its parents. Once the Heart has the necessary discipline, a child will be self-disciplining, and no longer need the parents' input and control.

As parents, if you have done a good job, when the fourteen-year-old feels his or her Liver flowering and opening up, his Heart will have the self-control to resist some of the more outrageous suggestions that the Liver makes to it. If the child's Heart is poorly disciplined and has poor control over its subordinate organs, it will not control the Liver's urges to swear, rant and rave, or strike out violently etc. If this discipline is not learned before 14 or so, and learned from the parents, then it is very difficult to learn in later life..

At 15-16 years old, a child becomes fixed in its patterns of Qi and it is at this time, the last of the organs come into the cycle, namely, the Kidneys. The Kidneys, up to now, have been making the body. The body has been growing in height, complexity and strength. At about 16, the body is usually almost adult and the Kidneys can rest more often and growth is much slower for the next three to four years. The Kidney therefore can spend more time giving energy to its other functions, such as a lust for sex and dealing with fear. Fearlessness is unparalleled at any other time of life.

What happens if the Heart is poor at controlling the other organs? When energy is low for some reason, the Stomach will ask for energy in a form that gives a quick response, rather than a form that requires the Stomach to work hard to get the energy.

Here's an example:

"STOMACH": "How about some chocolate?"

"HEART": "Ok, but send some of the energy to me."

The poorly disciplined Heart therefore attains some energy, short lived as it is, from the Stomach. As the Heart is responsible for happiness, the person feels slightly happier for the chocolate. Some may call it a wicked joy.

The correct Heart response of course is: "No, we need food that will sustain us".

Therefore the Stomach will have to work harder to break down the food, but will obtain more and better energy from the effort. The energy will also last longer and produce better effects on the whole body. The Heart however, whilst benefiting in the long run and becoming overall a better and more balanced organ will not obtain the quick fix, short lived peak of joy. It is no wonder that poorly disciplined teenagers are attracted to powerful drugs, alcohol and cigarettes. The Heart knows intellectually that these things are wrong, but for a quick buzz, and a short lived joy fix, they allow the other organs to dictate wants and lusts over reason and logic.

At 13 or 14 years old, the Liver is strong and wants to be angry all of the time, and even violent. If the Heart is poor at controlling the standard organs that it knows already, a new one, like the Liver, is very poorly controlled, if at all. At 16 years old, when the Kidney comes on line, the child is no longer fearful of consequences and is interested in sex. It is then extremely important for the Heart to have and exercise control. If you do not exercise discipline over the 5 year old child, then the 16 year old adult will not be able to discipline him or herself and may, if socially unacceptable, go to jail or worse.

One thing is certain, if the problems are not corrected before 16 years old, they are less likely to be repaired after this time. A person is capable of altering their behaviour to become more socially acceptable, but it will always be a veneer, and the adult will never be deeply in control of himself or herself. If you want to see a person's true nature, deprive them of sleep, and their ability to cover up their personality traits will be seriously reduced.

The first 5-8 years of a child's life are vital for their future personality.

CHAPTER FIVE

Birth with Acupuncture

When a woman becomes pregnant, she has a baby inside her which is dependent on her for its life. The word 'life' is used in its fullest sense, not just chemicals passed in the blood, but all of the requirements for life, such as emotions, movement, stimulus, energy and contact.

As we will see later in Relationships (Chapter 23), every person's personality produces a Qi pattern around them. To put it more correctly, the internal organs of a person generate a certain Qi make-up, which produces or controls the personality, as well as a Qi field around them, sometimes called an aura.

This aura interacts with other auras to produce relationships, likes and dislikes or in other words, our reactions to other people. The strength of the response is due to: a) proximity, and b) the strength of the organs most involved. Consider two pairs of cogwheels. The first pair has very small teeth. The wheels can come quite close together before one impacts on the other, and makes it run in sequence with it. If the teeth mesh well, they will spin about together in relative harmony but it is easy for them to separate as it takes only a slight shift away to disengage the teeth.

If the teeth do not mesh and are not compatible, they will have little effect on each other and will only affect each other when very close together.

These wheels represent mild or orthodox personalities. They run with the crowd, have nothing extraordinary about them and do not upset anybody, or at least very few people. It is not hard for them to alter slightly to fit into any group or community, and they need other people. They are good citizens and need to be one of the gang. They get lonely easily and when they move or travel, they become a part of the new scene quickly.

On the other hand, if the wheels have some large teeth, and some small, the effect on other wheels is felt at a greater distance. Also, there is a distinct disharmony if the wheels close by cannot accommodate their eccentricities. When this type of person finds a cogwheel that can spin with it, without too much bumping and grinding, it is a spectacular and special relationship. People represented by this type of wheel are loners, and form few, but strong relationships.

What does this have to do with babies? When a mother is pregnant, her baby has potentials that have been predetermined at the time of conception. From then on, the mother's Qi pattern, or aura is influencing baby. With all this Qi pattern influence, the baby comes out as close to the mother's pattern as possible. Given that the genetics of the baby are different to mum, baby's Qi pattern is similar but will change later.

The similarity is necessary, as once born, the baby is going to have to be close to and be nursed by its mother, and cannot be abhorrent to the mother, even if the father is, and even if the child grows up to become that way. At birth, the baby is as close as possible to a copy of mother's personality. Some genetic makeup will show up whilst inside the mother if the father's influence was strong enough at conception. The baby will also have some effect on its mother's personality during the pregnancy. This is not the cause of the mother's personality change when pregnant. The mother displays signs of being pregnant, due simply to the fact that she is pregnant. Most of the change in the mother's personality is due to blood deficiency.

To make a baby, the mother has to feed it blood. The baby needs blood to live and survive. But mostly, it is blood that provides all of the building blocks that build a body. Not only that; all the waste produced from a living, fast growing body is transferred to the mother's blood to be disposed of. It is no wonder then, that the mother presents signs and symptoms of blood deficiency and hot, poisoned blood. These symptoms of blood deficiency include: hair falling out, pulled tendons, sore joints, dizziness and fuzzy thinking. The emotions are dulled and not felt as strongly and the brain does not seem to think as clearly. Thoughts are not as sharp and clear as they would be if the blood volume was up. Hot blood produces rashes and itchy feelings. Some women even suffer from candida albicans.

Also, early in the pregnancy the Stomach gets too hot and rebels, resulting in nausea and sometimes vomiting. Another sign of a hot Stomach is the propensity for conversation, especially about themselves.

During the entire pregnancy, the mother must be on her guard against blood deficiency, as well as maintain a good quality of blood. Luckily, if there is a problem with the blood volume, then only the mother is affected by the problem and the system makes sure that baby is well supplied. There has to be severe blood deficiency for baby to be affected. If the baby is suffering from a short supply of blood, then the baby's body, nervous system and organs will be underdeveloped and immature at birth. If there is a problem with the quality of blood, this is unfortunately a systemic problem, and both mother and baby are affected. The baby's growth and potential are both compromised if blood quality is poor.

So how do you make blood?

Blood volume is controlled by the amount of fluid you drink You cannot make blood from dry biscuits. Also, blood is hard to make, if you drink lots of cold water and drinks, this cools off the Stomach. The Stomach's job is to make blood from the fluids you drink. If the Stomach is cold and constantly filled with freezing cold water, it will not make blood, just urine.

Judicious drinking of room temperature or hot fluids will ensure an adequate supply of blood.

Food influences and controls the quality of blood and what goes into the blood, but again, if the Stomach is filled all the time, it cannot supply the rest of the body with energy, and it cannot transform food energy into blood goodness. Food has to be eaten judiciously and only when the Stomach is able to process it properly. If the Stomach cannot process the food, it is simply sent down to be eliminated. When you have bowel motions that are smelly and have undigested food in them, it means that the Stomach has not been able to take the goodness out of the food. If you are passing undigested food, this is a waste and damaging to the Stomach.

During the last few weeks of the pregnancy, the mother's body begins to build up lots of blood. The blood is stored and held near to the baby so that when the birth process is underway, it all goes smoothly. The mother's muscles will need lots of blood for when they open up for the baby's passage. Lots of blood will be required for the lubrication of the birth canal, and lots of blood will be required for the womb muscles, for their effort in pushing baby out. The whole process of birth is dependent on an adequate supply of blood. If the blood volume is full, then birth will proceed smoothly.

When an acupuncturist attends a birth, his first diagnostic examination is to check the colour of the fingernails, face and tongue. These are the tell-tale signs of the amount of blood in the body which will give a good indication of how hard the birth will be and how much work the acupuncturist needs to ask of his needles. If the blood is deficient, it will probably be a long night, and the birth will be slow. Even acupuncture will not do a great deal of good, because blood cannot be made whilst in labour. Fluids can certainly be supplemented, but not to any great extent. However, if the acupuncturist has been consulted throughout the pregnancy, the blood will be full, and the birth will come at the right time, with little trouble or intervention. The acupuncturist should therefore not be required at birth . If the acupuncturist is called because the birth is proceeding poorly, the job is usually hard, due to the lack of blood. This does not mean that it is impossible, or that the needles cannot assist even the most hopeless cases. But the quantity of blood in the mother is directly related to the efficacy of acupuncture during birth.

In Chinese medicine, pregnancy seems to approximate "lower heater damp accumulation". It seems reasonable therefore, that the points most effective for lower heater dampness, are those points used to induce labour.

The ability of the womb muscles to push the baby down is dependent on the Spleen, and how well it controls and tones the muscles, so points on the Spleen channel generally control the rate of contractions.

The dilation of the cervix is controlled by the Kidney yang, and Kidney yang points can assist the dilation if it becomes a problem, or is not dilating.

Transition is the period where baby wants to be pushed out, but the mother's body is not yet ready for the second stage, so confusion of the body and mind occurs. This is a Heart problem and Heart points can be used to provide a smooth transition from the 1st to 2nd stages.

After birth, if the mother has torn, usually the yang point of Kidney will stop or dull the pain while stitches are administered, together with Lung 7. If the placenta is not keen to come out, then the 'Womb Point', together with Spleen 6, can sometimes persuade it to do so.

Sometimes, if drugs have been used, as well as the effects of a small amount of alcohol, bleeding internally can be a problem. Chinese medicine assigns this to reckless and hot blood, and the blood points Spleen 10 and Bladder 17 are used, together with some "White Powder" herbal formula, which most acupuncturists carry about, and which is known far and wide as a "bleeding stopper".

CHAPTER SIX

Early Childhood

At the moment a baby is born, it is said that the Lung channel commences operation. Up until this point, there has been little need for normal Qi meridians to flow, due to the smallness of the body, and the proximity of the mother's Qi surrounding and nourishing the baby.

However, at birth, the absence of the mother's Qi makes the Lung meridian open, and the Lung organ begins to work.

When the Lung organ starts working, it feeds air energy to the Lung meridian and asks for the Stomach to supply food energy, and therefore, the baby breathes and looks for food. This way, the Stomach organ can take energy from the mother's milk, the Lung organ can take energy from the air and mix these two energies. The Lung then feeds the Zong Qi, or chest energy into the Lung meridian at the acupuncture point Lung 2 (or some say Lung 1). This energy now called Zhen Qi travels down both arms and makes the arms work, which is why most babies' arms will wave about in the air before their legs move.

This energy travels back up the arms via the Colon meridian and from there into the Stomach meridian, as the Stomach organ needs to be fed with Qi, so that it can digest the milk. The Stomach meridian then flows down from the Stomach organ and into the front of the legs, and you will see baby kick his legs forward in response to this. The Qi will generally not be sufficient to go beyond this point and it is rare to find a baby whose Qi is able to flow up the body and into the Spleen organ. Luckily, for the second period of life (gestation being the first), the baby does not require any further organs. The baby only has to eat, breathe and remove waste.

After some weeks, a small amount of Qi reaches the Spleen and some muscle tone is provided, together with a little cognition. Memory of a type is also available. The Spleen doesn't really come into its own until about 4 or 5 years old. Very few people can recall what they did before 4 years old, and a strong Spleen organ gives you the ability to recall. If the Spleen is weak, then it will not be capable of recalling many things. If it is strong, then the memory will be considered strong.

With some meditation techniques and hypnosis, all organs, including the Spleen can be modified and tonified, usually at the expense of another. Also, as the Heart gains control of other organs, it tells those organs what to do, and in the case of the Spleen, how much it is to remember. Hypnosis and meditation remove the influence of the Heart, and access the organs directly. This can be extremely useful, or can be somewhat harmful. There are often very good reasons why the Heart has told the Spleen to forget certain events. Sometimes there are not.

The Qi rises up the leg in the Spleen channel into the Spleen organ and from there to the chest. As the Lung becomes stronger and pushes the Qi further, the Spleen channel turns into the Heart channel, and the baby's Heart becomes more active. At this point, the baby begins to control the Bladder and bowels. It can exert control over other organs and can combine with Lung to produce words, not just crying.

The main tell-tale sign of the Heart being fed with Qi (six to twelve months old), is that baby has the ability to laugh and giggle. It is important at this stage to instil discipline into the child. If discipline is instilled into the child at this stage by the parents, then the child's Heart will learn how to discipline and control the other organs. It simply learns by copying what it sees and experiences.

If the Heart is not capable of control over the other organs at this stage, then it will be incapable of control over the stronger organs, once they begin to operate. Self-control exerted by the child is simply the child's Heart organ exerting control over the other organs.

In the West, we say the same thing slightly differently; reason should overcome base animal instincts for humans, especially the more civilised, cultured and educated they are.

The two similar situations below show the importance of this system.

A young 3-year-old lives on a side street, very close to the main road. Reason, logic and consequences are, as yet, not available to the young 3-year-old. His mother tells him not to run out into the road. Yet he sees Mum and Dad walk across the road on a number of occasions.

The young 3-year-old sees a red thing on the other side of the street. Thinking of nothing else, and not having any self-preservation energy, he begins to cross the road. Mum is standing next to him at the time, and pulls him back. If she does not discipline the child immediately, then the child will not learn to obey its emperor (Heart) under all circumstances. If this is not instilled, then one day, when the mum is not about, the toddler will walk out onto the road and possibly be injured or even killed. Reason and logic don't apply. The toddler must be made to do what he's told, or his internal make up will not comply with the "Universal Pattern of Nature". When the Heart is controlling the child, the base emotions, (i.e. other organs), will be kept in their place. Whilst their job as ministers is to give advice from their own points of view, the king, or Heart is required to consider all advice and make a judgement accordingly, not to be bullied into it.

Our second situation is when a person jumps into the water. His head goes under the water, and stays there. Consider the organs fighting amongst themselves.

The Lung says, "I want to breathe, open the mouth so I can breathe". Spleen is the memory, and tells the Heart, "When you are in water you cannot breathe, remember last time"? Therefore, the Heart tells the Lung it cannot breathe just yet. As time goes by, the Lung becomes insistent, and complains that if it does not breathe the Qi flow will stop, but the Heart remains adamant, and together with the Spleen and Stomach tries to reach an air source. If this is not done, the Lung organ cannot send Qi to the body, especially the Heart, and consciousness ceases, then finally so does the brain, Heart etc., and death occurs from a lack of oxygen.

Now, if the Heart is not strong enough, then the Liver organ will make its presence felt, and the Heart will not stop it from insisting that the Lungs take a breath. Then panic ensues, due to uncontrolled fear. A person's ability to control the instincts of the normal organs is assessed from the person's Heart, and how much influence it holds over the other organs i.e. how much discipline was instilled into the child before the powerful fire organs (Liver, Stomach and Kidney Yang) were old enough to exert influence over a weak Heart.

CHAPTER SEVEN

The order in which our organs grow up

If you ask a Western medical scientist which organs are operating in a healthy child at any given time, they will assure you that they are all working. The traditional Chinese view is slightly different. Whilst the physical organs must be operating, some are not at full capacity and are carrying out their jobs at different rates. As TCM bases its understanding on symptoms, then some organs are not fulfilling all of their functions. In fact, from conception to four years old, there are only limited meridians and acu-points on the body. Baby anatomy from a TCM point of view is different. (Tiquia, R. *Chinese Infant Massage* Melbourne: Greenhouse Publications)

The Chinese count age from conception, so that at birth, a person is nine months old already. For convenience, they usually just add one year to anyone's age. When they say five years old, they are usually talking about someone we would say was four years old.

Throughout this whole book I have used Western ages, and will continue to do so. In TCM terms, life begins at conception. The foetus is growing during pregnancy and therefore subject to

Kidney energy, and Spleen energy. The Kidney builds the bones and brain, and the Spleen builds the flesh. These organs have such a huge job to do that they cannot do all of their other appointed tasks. From the outside many functions appear to be inoperative.

At birth, many things happen. Firstly, the Lungs have to operate, both physically as well as energetically. As the Lungs begin their 90 or 100 year journey, their energetic influences also begin.

The Lungs take energy from the air and send it into the Lung meridian. It is no surprise then that the Lung meridian is the first meridian in the sequence of meridians. The Lung also controls the skin. Now that baby is out of its cocooned existence, it needs an immune system on its skin, to keep it healthy. The Lung controls Wei Qi, (protective Qi) on the skin.

The Lung also controls its yin/yang partner organ, the Colon. Not long after breathing begins, the Colon makes its first movement.

The Lung and Colon are not enough to support the baby, and another organ begins soon after birth. This is of course the Stomach. The order of the meridians in sequence is: Lung, Colon, and Stomach. Human beings take energy from food by using their Stomach, send this to the Lungs, and the Lungs take air Qi, and then mix these two types of Qi together. The Lungs then send the mixed air and food Qi into the meridians, which sustains life. The Lung and Colon then remove the unwanted and waste parts of the air and food respectively.

At about one year old, a baby begins to talk. To do this, Heart energy is required, that is, logical sequences of thought. Whilst the Heart (the physical organ) has been pumping blood around the body for a long time, and the person's spirit has been residing in the Heart since well before birth, the signs and symptoms of the Heart have been hidden. The sequence of Qi flow in the meridians follows from Lung, Colon, Stomach, Spleen, to Heart, and Small Intestine. With Heart and Small Intestine now "on line", the baby can accept and process new ideas, form logical chains of thought, and understand and replicate sentences. A baby can even have unique thoughts.

Around twelve months later, growth slows down a little and some of the Kidney energy is channelled into the Bladder, and this allows the baby to be potty-trained. The Bladder controls the collection of the urine, and the Kidney yang is in control of the sphincters, both front and back. And yes, the Bladder and Kidney meridians follow next in the sequence.

The Chinese have followed life changes in people for many years and have come up with the concept that males and females have slightly different life cycles.

Girls have a life change every seven years. So at about six years old, girls have a life change. Their Spleens become stronger, and they begin to exhibit Spleen signs. These signs include memory, concentration for lengths longer than three minutes, and muscle tone. The baby fat tends to slip away and some physical ability manifests. It's at this age that they can begin to train at some sport or musical instrument.

Boys however are slower in their development. They have an eight-year cycle.

This change generally happens to them one year later at seven years old. Their ability to learn at school is also one year behind. Boys change from being a baby to being a child one year later than girls.

As discussed in a previous chapter, the Heart comes on line at about one year of age. Before a baby can talk, it's almost impossible to spoil your child. After the Heart opens and is working, discipline should be administered. If the Heart can learn to control Lung, Colon, Stomach and Small Intestine, then when the Bladder begins to operate, the Heart can control this too. This is important for later, because the Kidney is also involved with toilet training. The Heart needs practise at controlling the other organs (self-discipline), because when the Spleen becomes strong, it also needs to be controlled. This practice of self-discipline has seven or eight years to become solid and well entrenched, before the next life change occurs.

At 13 for girls, and 15 for boys, the child turns into an adolescent. At this time, the Liver and Gall bladder, the last organs on the meridian chain open up in earnest.

The Heart needs to keep a control over these organs or they will overpower the Heart and cause gross, socially unacceptable behaviours. On the other hand, if properly controlled and used, the Liver energy can be channelled into a grand purpose.

Properly controlled, the Liver makes one dynamic, effective and a person who finishes what they start. Poorly controlled, one is quick to anger, regularly depressed and plans poorly. You may even over-plan all occasions, only to have your plans go wrong.

One or two years later, the Kidney organ, having mostly completed its work on building the body, will begin to develop other ways of expending energy. Kidney yin repairs damage, and Kidney yang lusts after members of the opposite sex. So teenagers tend to get into fights, where they are damaged and need to repair. They may begin to smoke or drink alcohol, whereby large areas of the body are damaged, and Kidney yin is required to be expended. They would be better served to get a part time job, or learn martial arts, or some other sport. Each time they damage themselves, Kidney yin is expended to do the repair, or to control the pain, and the Heart receives a charge of joy. For teenagers this makes them happy. It may also provide some explanation of the self-destructive tendencies so prevalent in some teenagers.

To expend Kidney Yang, they look for, talk about, think about, and sometimes even try sex, mostly by themselves, but eventually with others.

A measure of character, or adulthood, can be argued as the ability of the Heart to control the Kidney, Liver and all the other organs clearly, and totally.

To say it another way, your ability to exhibit appropriate amounts of appropriate emotion, at the appropriate time is your entry key to the adult world.

CHAPTER EIGHT

Heart is King –The Joy of Discipline

In Chinese medicine the twelve organs of the body are likened to the ministers of the government. During the times in history when Confucians ruled China, each area of China was ruled by a local governor, who reported to the governor of the province. The provincial leaders all reported to each of the eleven ministers who were responsible for various stems or parts of the kingdom. For instance, one minister is responsible for water, another for rubbish, another for war, etc. All ministers are under the control of the King, or Emperor. He allows each minister autocracy to a point, but the Emperor has the ability to oversee all eleven areas of concern and will overrule or control if necessary. Also, each minister reports to the Emperor regularly and on every major decision, they are all asked for input from their point of view. The state of the kingdom as a whole is judged by the quality of the Emperor. There were times when the Emperor was weak and was not able to control the ministers and they controlled the kingdom in an unbalanced and biased way. At other times, the Emperor would be conscientious and would strive to be the best Emperor that he could be, expecting and attaining the best from the ministers, who would attain the best from their underlings, right down to the local workers, striving to be the best workers that they could be. The kingdom was then strong, fair and easy to live in.

This is a Confucian model of government and is based on the Confucian model of heaven. In the Confucian heaven, there is God, who rules all of heaven. He has eleven ministers who report directly to him and control each of their particular portfolios. The lower angels and divine beings control their different areas, and so on, to the lowest personal guardians that we all have.

Confucian logic suggests then that a person's body obeys a similar pattern. The Heart is the King, or Emperor. If there was such a thing as a perfect childhood it would include a perfectly disciplined Heart which would then in turn discipline the other eleven ministers (organs) that report to it. These ministers have areas of the body that they control and administer. The Heart also has a small portfolio of its own. Mostly, this portfolio is of a supervisory nature. Heart has control over the deeper thinking ability, capacity for joy as well as sleep.

Take for example, the Lung's portfolio which is to oversee the flow of Qi and smooth operations. Therefore Lung looks after things such as; - smooth skin and hair, clear air passages and no coughs, enough self-confidence to progress through life's tough situations smoothly, and, with the assistance of its sister minister, the Colon, the smooth expulsion of poisons out of the body.

If the Lung does not receive enough air, the Heart has the ability to make the Lungs work better. However, when a person is underwater, the Lung's passion for air is a dangerous thing, it must be over-ruled by the Heart/King, who has an overall view of the situation and will not allow a breath until the mouth reaches the surface.

This continues to apply all through life and through all situations. Each organ looks after its own domain and the Heart must oversee from a height.

So if the Heart is hot and overactive, then the person's thinking will continue for longer than needed and this usually results in insomnia.

If you are tired and cannot sleep, cool the Heart. You can usually do this by cooling the Stomach with an ice block, or cooling the blood with cold water on the wrists. If the Heart is generally cold, then poor thinking, or foggy thinking results, together with a humourless disposition and constant sleeping. This problem is usually overcome by eating spicy foods and creating more heat.

People like this suffer from poor circulation and have pale to grey complexions. Some regular exercise and hot quality foods would help greatly. Foods that are hot in quality are foods like chilli, curry and spicy foods.

CHAPTER NINE

Children's Organs are not Solid

Have you ever played with plasticine, or perhaps moulded clay into a cup, then fired it? Children are like this. It is acknowledged by most people that upbringing influences children into becoming different types of adults. For instance, a child suffering with a tyrannical father will grow into a man who has difficulty being comfortable around older, stern men, even when middle aged.

It is further acknowledged that genetics play a role in forming the personality. Personality traits run through families for generations, as do certain types of physical features. The argument has raged in the West between nature and nurture for many years. As usual, somewhere in between is correct.

The Chinese way of viewing the world is to see the baby as having a personality of its own, with a collection of energy networks even before birth. At conception, the energies of the mother and father are given to the baby.

Once the pattern is set, the energy pattern begins to build a body, based on the available energy provided. The supply of blood in the mother's body has a bearing on how well the baby's body is built. Both the quality and quantity of blood are factors. But even the best fed foetuses cannot grow into a baby beyond the potential set down for it by the combination of parents' energies. A baby can, however be damaged by a poor blood supply, by a lack of supply, a lack of quality, or simply an excess of poisons.

Mothers who drink, smoke, take legal drugs or illegal drugs are not doing anything good for their babies.

On the other hand, once a baby is born there is some room for improvement. This is a most exciting and wonderful time for parents. They see their children with almost unlimited potential; they could be fire-fighters, or lawyers, or even doctors. The baby's potential is fixed, but by altering the organs at the right time, during childhood (the overall potential of the organs have not changed), but the external manifestations can be modified before the person's Qi pattern is set.

Some individual organs can be altered, both in strength and size. The idea is to mould the organs before they become set and immobile. Whilst this is good from one perspective, it is a double-edged sword as well. If a child's energy patterns are disrupted during childhood, once their organs are fixed, there is little that can be done to alter them. This does not mean that adults (over 21 years old) cannot alter their personalities, but it is very difficult and takes a great deal of effort. Usually the change does not work very well, or for very long. The old proverbs of "old dogs" and "new tricks", and "a leopard cannot change its spots" hold true most of the time.

But children can be altered and moulded easily and usually permanently.

Let's take the example of self-reliance. When a child is brought up to be self-reliant by its parents, the teaching is slow but consistent. There will certainly be some innate self-confidence due to the quality of the Lung energy.

Self-reliance must be taught by way of praise when demonstrated, and dissatisfaction when not. This praise and dissatisfaction by the parents can be feigned as well as actual. On the other hand if the parent is intent on the child having little self-reliance they will discourage these attributes when the child exhibits them. Therefore a child's parents can manipulate personality traits simply by demonstrations of praise or dissatisfaction at appropriate times. Once the child has a fixed habit of exhibiting these personality traits, they will use them with ever increasing skill. If these traits are still consistent at puberty, then the pattern and personality trait will remain for the duration of adulthood.

If a personality trait that the parent is trying to help the child establish is difficult to build, then another method for promoting it, is the use of example. If the child sees the parents or other adults that it respects successfully employing and using these personality traits, then it will make every effort to copy them.

62

CHAPTER TEN

The Finger Vein – A Diagnostic tool

Young Children are a worry. When they are sick, you don't know how bad they really are.

A young child has no experience to call on and cannot give you any indication of the severity of the problem. During the Ming Dynasty (1368-1644 AD), the Chinese began to use infant massage as a distinct therapy, as opposed to the usual herbs and acupuncture. One of the techniques of this therapy is diagnosis using the finger vein.

Children cannot talk very well before the age of about twelve to eighteen months, and after that they tend to be uncooperative in clinic. Any information that you receive will be from observation or from the mother or father. This can occasionally be misleading and subjective. The ancients found a simple test to use on children, which gives an accurate guide to the severity of a disease.

This system can be employed by parents as well as doctors, and will quickly and simply show the depth of the disease. Each of the index fingers has a blue vein that travels from the tip to the palm. This vein can be seen clearly on the edge of the finger where the white skin meets the red skin. In children above five, and in adults, the skin is too thick and the vein may not be visible, even when sick. On the other hand, in children under five, their skin is usually quite transparent, and the vein will give a good indication of the disease.

Take one of the index fingers of the child and give the area around the skin colour junction a rub, usually against the flow of the blood (towards the tip of the finger). If they are not sick at all, the blue vein will be clearly seen on the palm of the hand. If, on the other hand, a disease has entered their body, they will have the blue line crossing into the first joint of their finger. This means that the disease is in their Qi or energy. This is not a serious disease. But it will warrant a day off school, or a careful eye on the type of food eaten. Generally with children, a day in bed will relieve this type of disease.

If you find that the blue line extends into the middle third of the finger, then the disease is in the blood, and this is a more serious disease. With this indication, parents are well advised to seek medical attention, either from a Chinese medical practitioner or from an alternative practitioner, such as a naturopath or a Western doctor. The section from the last joint to the tip of the finger is the area that should concern most parents. This is the 'Ming', or 'life' area. If the blue vein can be clearly seen entering this part of the finger, you should be consulting a Western doctor quickly. A Chinese practitioner will also assist, and if possible both should work together. Do not be misled by a friend saying that their child had something similar, and it turned out to be nothing. A disease in the Ming will not easily go away, and the child may have the problem for a long time, perhaps for twenty years. I have seen some asthma sufferers with this indication, and if the problem is not attacked properly the asthma will follow them all of their life, rather than only at various times in their life.

If you become proficient at this type of diagnosis you can start to compare the two sides of the child. The finger vein on the left hand is indicating the blood side of the body, and the right side is the energy or Qi side. This means that the diagnosis can be even more accurate by a simple comparison of the two sides.

CHAPTER ELEVEN

Moulding an appetite

At birth a baby has no ability to digest food and needs sustenance from its mother. The mother has a system whereby the food she eats is digested and then made into milk, which gives the baby all of the nutrients it needs, as well as some of the microbes and antibodies (immunities) that it will need for its life next to its mother. As the baby begins to need more nutrients than the mother can supply, it begins to seek other food (solids). During the latter part of the first six months, the baby should be experimenting with tastes and foods. This generally comes with the ability to manipulate items into its mouth.

During the six months to two years stage of development, a baby has to learn to seek out food, and feed itself. Obviously it cannot do this at six months old but will begin learning this about that time.

This means that instead of just eating everything that is put into its mouth by mother, it will begin discerning tastes and refusing some foods. A wide range of food should be presented to baby at this time, and the baby's reaction to each food should not be recorded. In other words, if the baby refuses to eat a certain breakfast cereal today, this does not mean that you should not offer it again on some other occasion. There are a high percentage of mothers, who find the foods that their baby will eat, and then feed only them to the baby. Pretty soon there are only a few foods that the baby is inclined to eat all of the time. Also, there are those who will present the same food in a different format and then feel superior because they have fooled baby into eating what mum or dad feels will be good for him, whether it is correct or not. It's a good bet that if the baby ate it, it was what the baby wanted to eat anyway. At this stage, the baby is learning to eat and to taste, and needs to practice. Those foods that do not supplement baby's energy at that moment are rejected, and those that are good for him are eaten. On a different day, if the baby is in a different energy pattern, then he will eat different foods.

He should be given the opportunity to try.

On the other hand, up until two years of age, the baby also needs to develop a Stomach and intestinal system that can cope with some of today's foods. Foods should be experimented with, so that the baby can be exposed to a range of energies and microbes, some of which will live inside the baby's intestines for as long as fifty or sixty years. Whilst dairy foods are not usually suggested at this stage of life, some yoghurt for example is acceptable.

Until five years old, a baby generally has poor quality digestion. This can be seen from the quality of what comes out the other end and the difficulty with which a baby digests the harder to digest foods, such as dairy. In most cases, the best foods are the foods that are easily digested. These are the plain foods that are not full of flavour. Hot or spicy foods, or foods heavy in fibre are not generally expected to enhance a baby's digestion. The foods that a baby likes are those that are plain and mushy and well cooked, or even overcooked. These are the best foods for a baby until about five years old.

From five years to pre-teens these are the years that will determine the child's digestive system and to some extent their personality for the rest of their lives. If their digestion is too aggressive they will have personalities to match, and will be plagued by ulcers in the future. On the other hand, if they have a slow digestion they will suffer academically. As in all things Oriental, the middle way is seen as the best way to go.

During the pre-teenage years, children need a deep discipline instilled into them by their parents, so that their self-discipline will be moulded and shaped into a strong force that will work for them in their future. The Heart is the King and it is the organ that is responsible for discipline. The Heart is taught to be strong by copying the control exerted by the parents whilst applying this control over its own organ subjects. As usual, if the control by the parents is excessive the Heart learns wrongly, and a closed, withheld personality is the result. If the parents are too easy on the child, then the child is willful and the adult is far too subjected to the whims of the other organs since the Heart cannot control them very well, just as the parents could not control the child very well.

One of the big influences in this area is the debate on food. A child cannot have total control over its food intake. Mainly because it cannot select food well enough to ensure it receives the correct foods. On the other hand, if the parents do not allow the child to select some foods and make mistakes, then no learning will be done. The parents should point out any mistakes made by the child of course, and the learning will continue. This is usually what happens in most Western countries but if the parents know little about the foods that they are eating, they cannot give their children a lot of guidance. In many cases, the foods that they ate at the same age are totally unavailable, or have been altered by modern preparation methods. Furthermore, many parents forget what it was like and think that their children should have the same tastes as they do now. It usually does not occur to them that their present tastes are the result of years of trial and error.

It is only in the West that we seem to believe that children should think and behave like adults and that adults of all ages should think and behave the same. This is not the case, and if people are constantly changing their tastes and thought patterns, then their personalities are also changing all of the time.

If a pre-teen child is consistently using a hot Stomach to deal with the world, then he will be the type to crave for foods that cool the Stomach. You might see him drinking a litre and a half of milk for breakfast, and the same again after school. This will have the tendency to cool the Stomach and make him feel better. In the long term, this will produce the effect of making the Stomach used to dealing with milk and it will be constantly up, and hot, ready to deal with the large quantities of milk that it is expecting to encounter every day. On the other hand, if the child is not subject to a hot Stomach and drinks a lot of milk, the dairy will cool the Stomach too much, and the Stomach will struggle to digest food and may produce phlegm.

In the long term, the Stomach will be damaged and think that the correct state of affairs will be to be cool and not digest very well. From this you can see that milk has long term effects and short term effects, and both can be good or bad, depending on the type of child. One of the best judges of this will be the adult parent, who can make suggestions because they are probably of a similar type of personality, and they have already learnt what milk does to them. The concept that milk is bad for everybody is foreign to Traditional Chinese Medicine.

On the other hand, a curry or chilli type spice in the food will cause the Stomach to rise. If the child is quiet, introverted and withdrawn, then the idea of spicing the food will possibly appeal to them. If this is done on a regular basis the Stomach will begin to show changes, and will start to produce a slightly more extroverted child.

However, if the Stomach is already hot, and the spicy food is introduced on a regular basis, the Stomach will begin to expect it, and cool down overall.

This may be a good or bad thing, depending on where the child started.

CHAPTER TWELVE

Consolidation of Organs

Children are pliable. Their personalities are mouldable and changeable as they grow and learn. There is a certain amount of genetic imprinting and this is a biological requirement for the species. When a child is born it has an energy pattern that produces a personality and a physical body. There are potentials and capabilities that are fixed, but most can be altered, by damage, destruction or augmentation, and, as a foetus or newborn, the child can easily be damaged. As the baby grows older, it learns and this is the process of alteration of the basic genetic potentials. It can be taught socially acceptable behaviour, or unacceptable behaviour, and then builds on this behaviour as it learns further.

Let's take the example of Lung energy. From the above point of view, the baby may have inherited strong Lung energy. This energy allows the baby to cry and breathe well and in later life will give it self-confidence.

By constantly yelling at the baby or being irritated when it cries, the parents may reduce the Lung energy pattern because the baby learns not to use its Lung energy. This becomes acceptable behaviour for the household. As the child grows and leaves the household, even for short times, it will modify the behaviour, but the underlying structure will remain.

Conversely, if the baby has a Lung deficiency at birth, and has trouble breathing and crying, then the parents usually tell everyone and the baby how wonderful it is for not crying much, even when it has a dirty nappy. They give it plenty of sympathy, knowing that it has trouble breathing. The family doctor may diagnoses asthma. If this Lung energy deficiency is addressed before the age of 5, then the "asthma" should not recur for sixty or seventy years. On the other hand, if the child is given medication that damages the body, that reinforces the emotional pattern of being "asthmatic", then the Lung energy will continue to manifest this pattern.

Perhaps the most difficult task of parenting is to get the balance right between socialising a child to suit the family preferences throughout its childhood and thinking longer term to what is going to assist the child to grow into its full potential. To some degree, a child's Qi pattern can be manipulated to produce a body and a personality that is suited to what the parents want. So long term thinking is important. What may bring peace to the household at age ten may result in a failed job interview at twenty-one.

Cultural differences also add difficulty both in terms of time and place. If allowances for these factors are neglected, parents can find that their child grows up to be something that the parents don't understand, because they are from a different time and grew up in a different place.

Just before puberty, the Qi patterns start to become solid. The personality and body of the child becomes fixed and they are a lot harder to alter. It is then that parents realise that the unsociable behaviour that the child was displaying at age five, which was then considered cute, at fourteen, is embarrassing, and they try to change it, but it's too late. In the case of Lung deficient asthma, the child begins to use the energy of Liver and Kidney to overcome the Lung deficiency, and the doctor tells them that they have now grown out of their asthma. As soon as the Liver or Kidney energies are overstressed, it will return. This again alters their personalities and in adulthood they tend to exhibit Liver and Kidney deficient personalities.

At the end of puberty, the adult emerges after learning all of their childhood lessons and is ready to enter the adult world.

In this world, the adult is not shielded from the trials and tribulations of the real world (the way a child has been), and has to have a fixed Qi pattern, so that they are not unduly influenced by the big bad world. They can in fact make their mark on the world and change things for the better. If they are influenced too much, they will simply fall into the patterns that society decrees and not agitate for change. It is the process of sending out adults that have solid personalities who can think for themselves which is the cause of diversity and improvement in society.

CHAPTER THIRTEEN

Predicting Future Talent

One of the dilemmas parents face is what they should do about their child's future. If they are to go into a particular area or field of study, it should begin early. But what if they are not cut out for this particular field? There are three methods which may indicate a child's future talent.

The first method is history. A child will inherit certain talents and energy patterns from its parents. These talents and patterns not only come from parents but also from the method by which the children are brought up. It is therefore possible that a child will also inherit patterns and influences from grandparents, and other family members. When looking for future talents, you must find a common thread that runs through the occupations of its antecedents.

This should include parents, grandparents, uncles and aunts, cousins and other siblings.

The second method is to look at the body shape. In many cases the body shape can be improved by exercise, but there are certain things that are not influenced by exercise or the lack of it. The face is a good method to use for determining a future talent.

The first thing to look at is whether the eyes are close together or far apart. Close together means that they will be aggressive in their occupation and are suited to sporting fields and high stress administration occupations. When the eyes are far apart they are well suited to occupations where aggression is not praised or rewarded. An occupation such as teaching or working for large companies rather than working for themselves should be encouraged.

The third method to use is the ear lobe. This has been covered in Chapter 3, but is worth repeating. If the ear lobe is mainly close to the head then the person will have a large yin excess compared to the yang. These people generally think well and can spend long hours doing hard work at their desk. They should look at office work or at least at occupations where they can use their thinking powers for long periods of time.

If the ear lobe is away from the head then a yang excess will tend to manifest for their whole life. This type of person tends to age slowly, and is best suited to sports or outdoor occupations. At least they need to be physically active during the day.

UNDERSTANDING YOUR LIFE

A Patient's Guide to Chinese Medicine

Part Two

Adulthood

CHAPTER FOURTEEN

Sports Injuries

Sporting injuries can generally be split into two groups:

1) Blood deficiency problems.

2) Trauma or blood stagnation problems.

There is a third group, which we suggest is best dealt with by conventional Western medicine, which are those injuries where bones are broken or dislocated, or tendons and ligaments completely snapped. After the problem has been corrected by Western surgical means, a Chinese doctor may very well be able to help speed the healing to a certain extent, but will be unable to be of great help until the body is structurally sound.

Qi flows through the major pathways (meridians) in fairly well defined ways, that is, from fingertips to head, to toes, to body and so on. It is because these meridians have been plotted, that we're able to locate acupuncture points along them. While Qi flows through these pathways in a consistent manner, the person feels nothing. When Qi flow changes, there is a feeling.

For instance, when an acupuncturist inserts a needle, the Qi flow is usually disrupted from its present course. Sometimes it is slowed, sometimes sped up, sometimes sent backwards, sent deep or, at times just tonified or reduced. The associated feeling received by the patient is related entirely to how different the Qi pattern becomes, compared to how it was before the treatment.

On the other hand, if Qi is stopped, or altered radically, due to trauma, then the feeling will be quite severe. For instance, supposing you bump into the side of a table while you were walking around it. On your leg where the table hit you, the Qi will disperse. After a knock, the Qi disperses and runs away in all directions. This leaves the site of the trauma without Qi for a short time. At this stage the best treatment is to rub the site of pain, to try to return the Qi and keep the blood moving. When there is no Qi flow, the blood will not flow either. Therefore, what happens after the Qi disperses is that the blood will not flow, and it falls out of the meridians and into the flesh, stagnating there.

This is called a bruise. Over the next few days, the Qi returns, and flows through and around the bruise, slowly pulling the blood with it, so that it reduces in size and eventually goes away completely.

If your muscles use blood and Qi to do things, for example, physical work, then if you work too much, there will be a problem. As you begin your chosen sport or career, you will begin to use muscles in ways you have not done before. This will cause problems; the Qi will be used up and you will feel the muscle weaken and have less energy. If you channel more Qi to the site, eventually you will feel an overall weakness. We can call this tiredness. In addition, the available blood will be used up and more will need to be channelled in. In the end, you will find that small blood stagnations will be felt all over the muscle being used. In the West we call this lactic acid. They will be sore next day. This is Qi stagnation due to blood stagnation, caused by excess blood flowing into the muscles and unable to follow the Qi leaving. As no Qi is actually leaving the muscle, it is used up.

In small doses this is not a bad thing and the body copes by developing more Qi and better blood and Qi pathways, so that the next time this excess muscle action is required, the whole system will cope better. This is how a worker or sportsman builds their body to cope with what they need to do. If they do this gradually and continuously, with rest days, they can build themselves up into a professional (athlete or bricklayer, or whatever they choose to be).

However, when they train too hard, or don't have at least one or two days per week rest, they will tend to consume too much Jing. When Qi has expired, the body has a reserve system. It calls on the Jing from the Kidneys. This is acceptable occasionally, especially in the early stages. But if used to excess, too often, then the Jing channels will close down and not allow any more Jing to be used. This will lead to burn out or in some cases, chronic fatigue syndrome.

In most men, their blood levels are reasonably steady and their Qi levels go up and down daily. It is usually only in midsummer and midwinter when they forget to drink enough water, that they become blood deficient and begin to experience some depletion of blood. If they don't drink or eat properly, they will be prone to blood deficiency problems. The type of sports injuries experienced during these times will be those that occur late in the day, or late in the game.

Suppose you have played a normal first half of a game, and deep into the second half you feel a muscle, say calf or hamstring pull, and can barely walk off. This is a blood deficiency injury and can be avoided by drinking enough water and eating correctly.

Women, on the other hand, find that their energy use is usually consistent, but their blood goes up and down depending on the time of the month. It is extremely important for women to watch their periods to be sure that they do not develop overall blood deficiency. If the periods come late, or are short (less than two days), then you are in danger of overusing Jing. If the periods stop altogether, then you are, by definition, blood deficient and in a perfect position to damage muscles, tendons and ligaments beyond repair.

One more tip on sports injuries which may be somewhat controversial. In TCM we recommend, should you receive a blood deficient sports injury to muscle, tendon or ligament, not to use ice. Ice has the function of cooling and slowing the already deficient blood and although its benefits may be palliative, it will simply increase the area of damage, slow the recovery period and leave larger than necessary scar tissue.

CHAPTER *FIFTEEN*

Toes

Another method for diagnosing people and for understanding yourself is to look at the relative lengths and straightness of the toes. From the diagram below you can see that the toes have been labelled according to the organs that feed them.

During childhood, each toe is fed according to how much blood and Qi it receives down the meridian. If, during childhood a particular meridian is deficient, then that toe will grow to a lesser length than its full potential. The correct lengths for the toes are shown in the diagram. Each toe should be slightly longer than its outside neighbour. This should produce a straight line from the tip of the big toe to the tip of the small toe. The personality in childhood can be deduced from a close inspection of the toes. The left foot refers to blood and the right foot refers to Qi. Any left/right dichotomy can produce further insight into the personality.

If the toes are straight, then the meridian has been well nourished during childhood. On the other hand, if the toes are bent, or turned, then the meridian was affected. This can be from ill fitting shoes, as well as from inherited or learned Qi pattern anomalies.

Some toes are flat, and run almost exclusively along the ground, while some people have toes that rise where they attach to the foot, and then claw down to rest on the ground only on the pads. The first type usually indicates people who have relative yin excess, which pulls the toes down as they leave the foot. The second type have a relative yang excess, which pulls the toes up, and then nature pulls the toes down to the ground, as they are required for balance. This gives them a curved or clawed look.

Occasionally, you may meet a person with one clawed toe. You must look at which toe is clawed, or if the toes either side are flat.

Some people are pigeon toed and their yang is deficient. The yang is on the outside and pulls the foot out. If the yin is stronger, then the foot will point inwards. On the other hand, if the yin is deficient, and the yang is overpowering it, the foot will open out and the person will walk on the outside of their feet.

This may be interesting overall, but most diagnostic work is done through assessing the relative lengths of the toes. Here are some useful things to remember:

1) If the Kidney toe is very small, it can indicate a lowered ability to reproduce. These people may suffer an inability to have babies.

2) The Gall Bladder toe can reflect muscle problems. But mostly, if the toe is short and stunted, it can indicate that parents or circumstances thwarted their early attempts at decision making. They may thereafter suffer major frustration and will need to come to terms with this aspect of themselves as adults.

3) The middle toe is the Bladder toe. This reflects the hormone balance at puberty. If you find it too long, this may reflect an emotional upheaval at puberty, such as fear and insecurity. As a teenager goes through puberty, they are tossing their world upside down all the time. They need their home to be stable and consistent.

4) The second toe is the Stomach toe. If this toe is much shorter than it should be, you should be looking for a chronic disease of the Stomach.

On the other hand, if the toe is unusually long, or the tip is bent, then the person will usually suffer occasional bouts of hot Stomach, e.g. heartburn, stomach ache, and eventually a possible gastric ulcer.

5) People who have an abnormality of the big toe often suffer uro-genital problems. Also, the length and width of the toe can often indicate how much interest in sex these people will exhibit.

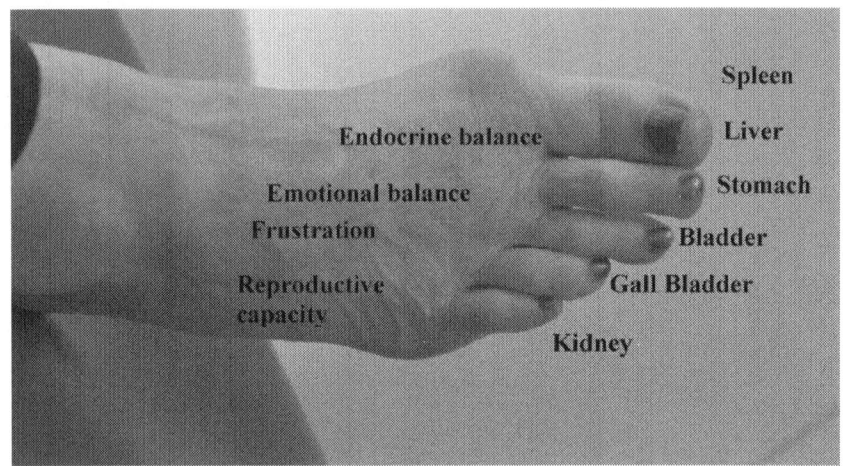

CHAPTER SIXTEEN

Sex Too Early

What happens when a child has sex too early in their life? The main focus of this chapter is the Kidney yang energy. Whilst Kidney yin determines the fluid regulation of the sex act, that is, when orgasm occurs, both in men and women, Kidney yang controls lust. The Pericardium controls the enjoyment of sex, or fantasies, but Kidney yang controls when these fantasies are to enter the consciousness and how often they are required to provide the Kidney yang's interest in sexual activity.

The normal maturing of a child into an adult includes a growth aspect that requires a lot of Kidney energy. Once the growth slows down and most of the bones are at a stable length, then the Kidney does not have as much work to do, and looks about for other activities. Often, at this stage, the teenager will seem fearless and will feel invincible. They may race cars, surf trains, or simply engage in lots of pub brawls and fights. Mostly, it is at this time when the young adult looks at procreation.

As usual, life is not as simple or as black and white as the model. Some people think of sex and feel lust well before they have finished building their bodies and should they engage in sexual activity they will cause damage to themselves. Should sexual activity be forced onto them, they will also suffer this damage. Most people see the psychological damage done in these circumstances, even in the adult, many years after it occurred. They do not always equate this with any physical damage. As we have seen over the last fifteen chapters, all problems have a physical and emotional side and you cannot have one without the other. Neither can you be mentally well adjusted if you are not physically well at the same time.

The best time of life to begin sexual activity is at a time when the organs, meridians and the psychological profile are solid and not subject to easy manipulation. The energy patterns of children are easily manipulated, whilst those of an adult are fixed and quite hard to change. Puberty spans both patterns.

If an adult has sex, it will alter their personality slightly, until the energy used can return to normal. Sex is a large drain of energy and can temporarily unbalance some personalities, or even rebalance some. For a child, the repercussions of sex will be overwhelming. The large drain of energy will leave a huge impression on the Qi pattern, and this alteration of the Qi pattern will not be to the benefit of the child in question. Generally, the adult suffers a temporary Kidney yang deficiency. With the child the Kidney yang may be permanently damaged.

Symptoms of Kidney yang deficiency include: low energy, introversion, sleeping a lot, no interest in sex, and no interest in sports or activities. This is not the only way that the Kidney yang can become deficient, so anyone exhibiting these signs has not necessarily been interfered with as a child.

A child's Qi pattern is not firm or solid, so after being interfered with sexually, they tend to have a hole in their Qi pattern, which will manifest in all of their later activities. The main (but not the only) disturbance of Qi for children that have been abused is the pattern of Kidney yang deficiency. Some children of course have received a Kidney yang deficiency pattern from their parents genetically, while others have had their yang disturbed by sickness or disease, or accidents.

When it comes to teenagers, having sex too early usually causes the opposite effect. If the young adult has a well constructed and solid Qi pattern, or (to say it another way) a well defined personality, then if they initiate their first sexual encounter they will usually enjoy it, want more and have their personality altered forever. This will not necessarily be for the worse. Often mothers and fathers will see the personality ripen and blossom after a teenager's first sexual experience. This can be a good and normal introduction into the world of adulthood. As a teenager, their ability to provide energy or Qi for the process is high, and the amount of Qi used will provide an enjoyable experience. Most sexual experiences from that point on will usually follow the same pattern and be enjoyable, while using a reasonable amount of Qi.

On the other hand, if the person grows up to save himself or herself for a marriage that happens too late and they are well into their late 20's or early 30's before they have their first sexual encounter, other problems may occur. Usually, the problem is that they do not have the "Ming Guan" ("Gate of sexual energy") open, and it tends to open only slightly after their first sexual encounter. Whilst they can engage in sex, and may even like it a little, they will never understand what all the fuss is about.

If a teenager is too young, that is, their personality is not solid and is able to be altered easily, they should not engage in sex. Leaving aside the problems with relationships and Qi flow between one person and another, there is also a real possibility that the Ming Guan will open too much, and will become too big, or remain open too much. This means that not only will the sexual act be really, really nice (due to the excessive amounts of Qi flooding the system), but the child will become what appears to be Kidney yang excessive. The personality will alter to: 1) cope with this excess Qi after every sex act, and 2) seek out further ways of obtaining more sex. In this case, sex becomes a drug and they become increasingly needful to keep their energy levels up and their entertainment up also. Each sex act also levels out their personality, so that they are psychologically very different before and after each coupling.

In the short term, sex becomes a drug and they are obsessed with it, due to the excessive flood of Qi into the system that accompanies it. By the time they reach their mid-thirties or early forties, they become Jing deficient, as they cannot sustain the excessive loss of Jing Qi every time they have sex. Despite their early training, they become Kidney deficient and sex becomes either unwelcome or unacceptable. They become angry and bitter, which results in difficulty holding friendships and relationships. This is basically burnout. There is little difference between this and a child suffering sports burnout. The Jing Qi costs to children when they over-train at their chosen sport are similar to the Jing Qi cost of having excessive sex. If the child is too young to have sex because it will devour large quantities of Jing Qi, then they are also too young to train excessively.

This brings up the obvious question: what if a teenager, who trains a lot, should begin indulging in activities that cost a lot of Jing Qi? Obviously there will be some serious consequences. The law requires that all persons be of a reasonable age, before they can legally have sex, drink alcohol, drive cars, smoke tobacco etc. There is good reason for this. Both Traditional Chinese Medicine and Western Medicine have come to the same conclusion on this matter. If minors entertain themselves with serious Jing usage, they will suffer long term problems because of it.

As a parent, your job is to see children into adulthood with the best personality and potential that you can, then leave them to their own life when they are adults.

CHAPTER SEVENTEEN

Alcohol

According to the "Jia Yi Jing" (265 – 420 AD), once alcohol enters the Stomach, the connecting vessels become full, and the normal meridians empty out. The result is that the alcohol floods its "impetuous and hot" energy into the skin and begins to damage the Stomach. This leads to the Stomach not being able to nourish the four limbs. If a person should repeatedly engage in sexual intercourse while drunk, or overeat while drunk, these will lead to heat in the interior, hot hands and feet, and a reddish colour in the urine. Because alcohol Qi is exuberant, impetuous, and aggressive, the Kidney Qi will debilitate daily.

Nonetheless, alcohol is used in Chinese Medicine for its ability to take the energy (Qi) of a plant or herb and place it into the meridian system quickly, without alteration. It is common for herbs like Ginseng to be stored in alcohol like rice wine, and when taken by the patient it is more effective because it enters the meridian system quickly, before the body has had time to alter it with digestion. Some herbs can be slightly nullified by the action of digestion, and are therefore less useful when finally absorbed into the meridians. Whilst this system of using wine is beneficial, there are those in the field who find that the negative effects of the alcohol outweigh the advantages.

In the field of Homoeopathy, practitioners also use alcohol to stabilize their homoeopathic medicines. This type of medicine is energetic and the stabilized energy pattern can be placed into the system quickly by following the alcohol into the meridians. The alcohol brings the pattern of energy with it as it passes into the meridian system. Which meridian it enters is subject to the individual.

After alcohol enters a vulnerable meridian, it quickly works its way into the associated organ and alters the organ's energy pattern. It does this in two ways. Firstly, the quality of the plant or herb that is mixed with the alcohol will alter the organ by imposing its Qi pattern on the organ. For instance, the herb or drink will do different things once inside. An alcoholic drink made from rice will have a different effect on you to one made from grapes, and a different effect to that made from cactus, or hops, or corn. Each of these will have their own quality of Qi pattern and they will impose that pattern on your organ. Your response will be different, depending on which organ is vulnerable, and how vulnerable it is. I have often heard people discuss the difference they feel between red wine and white wine. These differences will be due to the differences in the grapes that they are made from.

The second way in which the drink will affect you is via the action of the alcohol directly. In both Western and Eastern Medicine, alcohol is a poison, often used to sterilise. It will kill most if not all living tissue that it touches. When alcohol enters an organ, it affects the organ in the same way any other poison affects it. That is, it heats the organ and increases the yang content of the organ.

Now, there are five basic types of alcoholic effects that can be experienced by a person, as well as an infinite number of combinations. There are those that have a vulnerable Liver, and when they take drink, they experience a Liver yang attack. In other words, they will become angry, or violent, or depressed. Their reaction will be similar to any other Liver yang attack, but will be increased with the more alcohol consumed, and will ease if drink is not consumed.

Those people, who have a vulnerable Lung, will find that their self-confidence will rise proportional to the amount of alcohol consumed, and their voice will rise as well. These people tend to believe that they can do anything once they begin drinking. This can often be why they drink and they are often seen dancing on tables or lying in ambulances on their way to hospital after being involved in an accident caused by that very feeling of being invincible.

Some people have a vulnerable Stomach/Spleen complex, and when they drink, they become talkative. They almost always talk about themselves, and can be caught reminiscing about past achievements or failures. When they drink, other people think that they are a bore.

The Kidneys can be affected by alcohol if they are the vulnerable organs. The signs of an inflamed yang in the Kidneys are lustfulness or fearlessness. These people tend to become sexually available to a greater extent than normal. They are constantly talking about, thinking about and seeking procreation while under the influence of drink. The drunker they get the more they want it. Eventually, of course, as stated above, they become impotent and cannot have sex even when drunk.

Finally we come to the Heart organ. When alcohol affects the Heart, people will become introspective and deep thinkers. Their friends may consider them morbid and whilst their deep thinking may seem quite sensible to them, it is, in the light of day, somewhat moronic. This is because they have an artificial yang (thinking) Heart and the yin is lower than normal They will have a lot of thinking (yang), but their logic and sense (yin) are not available to control the thinking. After a reasonable amount of drink they will eventually fall asleep. This is due to the yin/yang concept of flipping from one extreme to the other. That is, if the yang becomes too excessive, it will flip over into a full yin condition. This is seen when a person gets too fiery, and they suddenly go very quiet and exhibit little fire.

The above scenarios may seem reasonable to the consumer because the artificial yang seems to be producing a better, all be it, short-lived, personality change. But the constant use of alcohol will have devastating effects. Here again Western and Eastern medicines begin to agree. After there has been consumption of alcohol, the body requires time to remove this poison and six to twelve hours (depending on health) is required to remove most of the alcohol. This means that the body is working on removing poison for most of this time. If you are a consumer of alcohol every twenty-four hours, then you can see that there are more hours in the day that you have poison in the system, than there are when you are clean. Even if you are drinking a small shandy every day, this is considered to be unhealthy in the traditional paradigm.

In Traditional Chinese Medicine terms, the aftermath of a drinking bout is dealt with by the application of Kidney and Liver yin. This yin is used to rid the body of the poison and requires time to recover. Usually a good eight hour sleep is the minimum. This is why you can wake dry, because the yin (fluid) has been used up. Sleep is not enough and fluid has to be enhanced all of the next day. If you cannot go all of the next day without a drink, then the yin will never be fully replaced, and depletion will occur. More importantly, the Jing will be used up. Jing is used to replace the yin that is not replaced by the normal processes of the body. This is much more serious, and as discussed in previous chapters, **Jing cannot be replaced.**

If the Liver is the organ that alcohol gravitates to mostly, long term drinking will see the Liver damaged. This will usually result in a fluid build up in the abdomen (ascites), cirrhosis of the Liver, or possibly permanent personality changes such as uncontrolled anger, or uncontrolled depression. One of the problems with the Western remedy for this is that allopathic medicines are dispensed, and these are dealt with by the body in the same way as alcohol. So the long-term problem is intensified, rather than repaired.

For those people where alcohol gravitates to the Lung, they are in danger of developing a cancer problem. Those people who drink to enhance their self-confidence are increasing the danger of getting cancer. Both Chinese medicine and Western medicine have evidence linking alcohol to the onset of cancer.

When the Stomach/Spleen is affected most of all by drink, long term drinking will usually lead to Stomach ulcers and unsociable behaviours. In the worst cases, these victims can be seen walking the streets, talking to themselves, often being unsociable to passers-by. They dress in rags, drink at any opportunity, are totally anti-social and talk constantly.

When the Kidney is the vulnerable organ and drink is used to increase sexual desire, the long-term result is impotence. In the case of women, frigidity. There is also a tendency to age early.

And finally, once again, we come to the Heart. Long-term drinking can lead to the Heart person suffering a stroke or Heart attack.

It is reasonable to reiterate that very few people will exhibit exactly the full quality of one organ, and not other organs. In other words, a person who drinks to excess will usually exhibit signs of two or more inflamed organs. For instance, those who inflame the Liver and Kidney will tend towards rage and lust, so rape is to be looked out for. Those who inflame Heart and Spleen will recount their days of old, until they drop off to sleep, still thinking that they are living in those bygone days.

Whether a person is a socially acceptable drunk, or a menace to society, the personality they exhibit is not real and is in all cases temporary. People who prefer their drunken personality should work to obtain it, not use a drug/poison to chemically manipulate themselves into it. This way ironically leads to the loss of the very qualities they are seeking, in the long run.

CHAPTER EIGHTEEN

Lines on the Face

Your body has been built by the energy pattern that supplies it with life. Because your parents gave you a certain pattern at birth (genetics), you built a body along those lines. All of your life experiences have altered the pattern of energy, and the organ balance has altered during life. You can, for instance, be provided with a genetic potential of being six foot six, and yet, through lack of nutrition, end up with a stature of only five foot ten. It then makes sense that if you are informed enough, you can read a person's life and experiences from what you see of their body. Many of the old texts describe what happens to a person when their Qi pattern is like this, or like that. When you see a person with one particular set of facial lines, you can confidently suggest that it is because of the person maintaining the pattern discussed.

One easy method to follow is of the lines on the face. Each line can tell you something about the person behind the face. Most people have discovered that to some extent they do this most of the time anyway. If you meet a person who looks like someone you know, you usually find that they have similar traits. Over years of experience you may find yourself holding preconceptions about people you meet because of the way they look, even before they open their mouth. It's not just whether they are tall or short, which is a common one, but also beautiful or ugly, red or blond hair, and my all-time favourite, smiling or gruff.

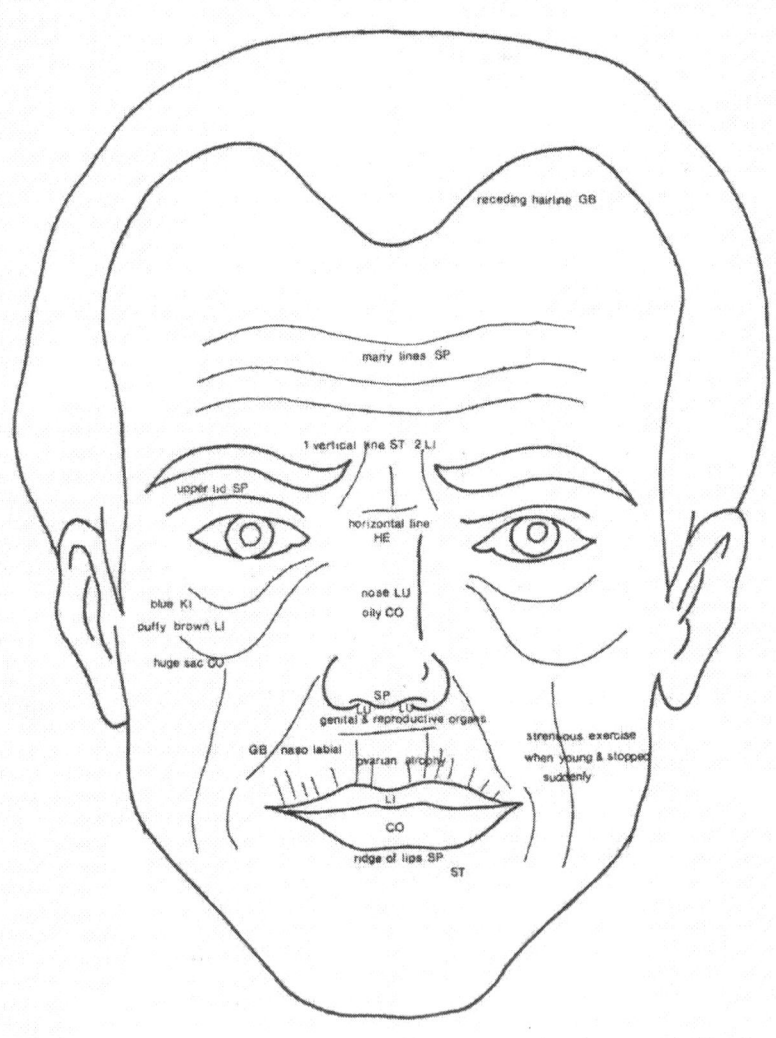

Over the centuries this face analysis has been recorded and those guesses that have proven to be correct most of the time have been maintained, and those that don't seem to work a lot of the time have been discarded. So now we seem to have a system that is fairly accurate, but always subject to alteration and of course in a world where Botox is increasingly available, there is more margin for error!

Let's start with some easy ones:

Colon: When the Colon has been working poorly, the bottom lip can appear to be too small, or too large. If the bottom lip is dry and cracked, the Colon is usually dry also. Other Colon signs are things like large bags under the eyes. Also, the nose can become oily and forehead headaches can be frequent. There may also be pimples on the chin. The Colon's job is to remove the waste from body, mind and spirit. Constipation can be an indication of a person's inability to let go.

Stomach: If a person has overused the Stomach, the forehead, just above the bridge of the nose receives a vertical line. This is one of the best indicators of long term Stomach overuse. As the Stomach rules the concentration, these people who have one line above their nose will handle problems with single-mindedness. Others might call them stubborn.

Liver: On the other hand, if two vertical lines appear above the bridge of the nose, just inside the eyebrows, then the Liver is the organ that has been most used by the subject. So, instead of using stubbornness to overcome problems they have tended to lean towards anger or depression. The other sign to look out for in the Liver arena, is the top lip. This can appear to be too small and many people know that this can be a sign of a quick temper. Liver's job is protection hence it translates well to the fight or flight response we speak of in the West.

Lung: Finally, a couple of signs that can be indicators of a Lung problem. The colour of the nose is significant as an indicator of the health of the Lung. Dry and gray is not a good look. Also, the whites of the eyes should be checked . If the sclera is a pure white, then the Lung energy is usually quite strong. But when the sclera has a blue hue, then the person you are looking at is possibly prone to a lack of self-confidence, and constant coughs, colds and even asthma. Lung is responsible for self-confidence and is sensitive to grief issues. From a Chinese medicine point of view, if we are grieving, it is akin to us saying "I cannot go on without you" which seen from a certain perspective is a lack of self-esteem.

CHAPTER NINETEEN

Sex

There are three things to consider and learn about sex, i.e. making love. There are three organs responsible for the satisfactory functioning of the body and mind while making love. Two of the organs are the yin Kidney and the yang Kidney. The yang Kidney, when not producing the fire for the Stomach to digest food, or not producing the energy for excessive sport, or excessive work, will produce the fire for lust. Kidney yang produces the fire that helps a person want to engage in sex. In men it is necessary in order for the act to take place. The physical act cannot happen if there is no Kidney yang raising the required apparatus.

For women there are less obvious signs, but a woman will definitely feel the yang rise. She can also feel the lack of Kidney yang when it is not available. The Kidney yang produces heat, and a person really does feel hot when aroused. Conversely it is difficult to become aroused if the person or people are in a cold environment. Outdoor rape is less common in the mid-winter time. The Kidney yang is busy keeping people warm, and there is not generally enough left for lust. Some exceptions do exist of course; such as when the Kidney yin is so deficient that even mid-winter is not enough to blunt Kidney yang's relative excess.

Therefore, if Kidney yang is lust, then Kidney yin is the ability to complete the act. In women it is the ability to orgasm. In men, it is the ability to keep the penis erect and to orgasm at will. Some men cannot control when the orgasm is attained, and this is a sign of low Kidney yin. If the Kidney yin is too weak then it is unlikely that the penis will stand up for too long.

Kidney yin's other functions are those of dealing with pain, repairing damage, and making fluid. It controls the strength of the knees and the lower back, as well as the emotion of fear. Some people may have experienced the effects of this; after sex of multiple types, or long sessions of love-making. They will feel weak at the knees, or worried about certain situations immediately after. After long periods of sustained sexual activity, often a sore lower back occurs. Often personalities change after long periods of unaccustomed sex and personalities also change after long periods of abstinence.

The third organ that plays a role in the sex act is the Pericardium. This organ is not a lot different from the Kidney yang, in that it deals with lust. Whereas the Kidney yang simply wants sex, the Pericardium deals with the enjoyment of sex, and how the act is performed. Some people like to be in bed, with the light off, some in public places, and everything in between. There are people who enjoy sex with their chosen spouse only, and others whose minds stray. There are as many combinations as there are people and it all comes down to what the Pericardium has decided is the most enjoyable sexual fantasy. If you refer to Chapter 8, where the discipline of the Heart is concerned, you can see that the Heart, and its ever present protector the Pericardium, need to be in control or else it can lead to trouble in later years. For teenagers who are starting out on the road to adulthood, the rules are simple: don't have sex with anyone you don't really like a lot, and don't have your first sexual encounter too early, otherwise you run the risk of suffering Kidney deficiency in later life.

For older people, sex can be a great comfort, but it can also ruin your health. "Moderation in all things", would be one of the most applicable sayings in this case. You cannot have sex as often, or as strongly as you used to, and you shouldn't try. Also, beware of your partners, especially if you don't know them well. Their lust or high Kidney yang may be keeping their personality balanced. Without this, they may become depressed or a layabout. Their Kidney yin may be the side that is up, and when this goes, their personality may become explosive, even dangerous.

Finally, you must be careful about how well they enjoy their sex. If you need to do a lot of extra to please them, you may end up with someone who needs a lot of strange and specialized methods of enjoying their sex. Discuss this early, so that you know what is pleasing to them and try to work out what forms this will take as the years go by. Also, do the same for your own particular needs. If you don't share compatible fantasies the relationship may be doomed from the start.

CHAPTER TWENTY

Heroes and Heroines

Who do you see as an heroic candidate? Who is your hero or heroine? Are they famous? Is it fame that makes them your hero? What are the criteria for being your hero?

In this chapter, I would like to offer a few ideas that you may like to consider. Traditional Chinese Medicine is silent on the subject, but traditional martial arts and traditional Chinese culture do share some thoughts about it.

A scorpion was running away from a bush fire one day, and came to a river. He ran up and down, and could find no way to cross the river. Suddenly, like a miracle he saw a frog in the middle of the river. He yelled at it, and asked him if he could carry him across the river. The frog came over, and looked at the scorpion. "If I let you on my back, you will sting me. That's what scorpions do". The scorpion explained that if he stung the frog, he would not make it over the river, and the scorpion would drown, as scorpions can't swim. This was logical and made good sense to the frog, and as it was a bush fire, most animals agree on a truce between each other till the fire is over and so he let the scorpion onto his back.

About half way across the river, the frog felt a mortal sting on his back and began to feel the poison flow into his body. He turned about and looked up at the scorpion. The scorpion had a fearful look on his face and knew he was going to drown. "Are you mad?" said the frog, "now we are both going to die".

"I know, but it's my nature, I couldn't help myself", said the scorpion and they both sank to the bottom of the river and died.

Was the scorpion simply subject to his own nature, and unable to control himself? As people, are we able to live better than that? Or is it impossible for "the leopard to change its spots", as many people believe?

Let's take the example of a student who is gifted at mathematics. He flies through school without a worry in maths and receives an "A" at the end of school. Is this praiseworthy? Compare this to the student who is better at English composition. At the end of their academic career, they end up with a "B" in maths only by a massive expenditure of effort and study. Which should receive more praise? Unfortunately, in the world as it stands at the moment, the wrong student will receive the plaudits.

How about the child, who is good at all sports and is top grade at three or four sports, then gives it all away, and becomes a slob? Contrast this to the child who has no aptitude, but practices like blazes and eventually plays a competent game of whatever game they choose to play. They play this game for many years and stay reasonably fit for their whole life.

What about the person whose Qi pattern has produced a personality that is a workaholic and because of this contracts Multiple Sclerosis? Instead of succumbing to this degenerative, life threatening disease, they change their personality and beat the disease. That's my hero or in this case, my heroine.

I have also seen and met people with cancer, who change their life and their Qi pattern so much that they can beat the cancer, and live a long and happy life, contrary to their nature. These people are worthy of high honours indeed.

So, if you are trying to bring up your children, are you teaching them to face their powerful and positive abilities with keen interest, or are you showing them that what they are no good at, they should avoid? Have you given them the example of trying hard to rid yourself of bad attitudes and habits, or the example of running from hard conditions, and putting up with your own inabilities?

If you have a constitution that is Liver dominant and are prone to outbursts of anger and violence, then make the effort to alter this by practicing patience. The more you can alter the pattern and remake yourself, the healthier your mind and body will be. If you are scared of aggressive people and physical contact, take up martial arts. If you are scared of water, take up scuba diving. If you have no musical aptitude, take singing lessons.

The people that inspire me are those who are doing things that are contrary to their nature. ***These people are heroes and heroines***.

CHAPTER TWENTY-ONE

Scars – Physical and Emotional

One day I saw a lady in clinic, who had a developmental problem. She had developed a body with large hips and thighs, and a small chest and small breasts. This was out of character with her family history both paternally and maternally. She asked me if Chinese Medicine had any reasons to explain why she had developed this way. The answer is an interesting one, and worth discussing.

Some time before she was thirteen years old, in her case eight, she had to have an abdominal operation. This operation was a success, and was without doubt required. But after the operation a large scar was left where the incision was made, across the lower abdomen. This meant that the meridians that flowed through this scar would be compromised, leaving the Liver, Kidney, Stomach and Conception vessels without a clear passage up the body. Whilst this lady was able to deal with a slight lack of Stomach meridian energy, her Kidney and Liver emotions were definitely compromised. Further, the Conception vessel is the control of yin climbing up to the head and also controls development. The simple answer to her question is that development was reduced after the scarring and the yin was excessive below the scar. This caused her to develop a pear shaped body, even though her genes were contrary to this shape. After the scar was treated, there was a slight shift in the Kidney and Stomach manifestations, but as the personality had been set and reinforced over many years, no great shifts could be made without a lot of personal effort from the lady herself. On the other hand, if I had had the opportunity to attend the little girl some years ago, she would have grown up as a different person, with a different body shape, and a different personality.

Why is this so? After the skin has been damaged, a scar forms. When you are a child, the Qi flows at a superficial level, just under the skin and any damage to the skin will receive the full force of the main meridians in its attempt to repair. Also, as children are full of Kidney yin, they tend to repair very well, and their scarring is usually small and full of energy. Even large areas of damage can repair well, with minimal scarring or scarring that looks a similar colour to the skin that surrounds it. This signifies that the Qi is flowing through it, rather than around it. If the damage is repaired well, the Qi will flow in and through it well, with little interruption. On the other hand, if the scar is formed at a time when the person is either Kidney deficient, or yin deficient, then the scar will form poorly, and Qi flow will be compromised. In this case, the main flow of the disturbed meridian will bleed into the surrounding Luo vessels (fine capillary type meridians), and try to find a way around the blockage. Over years, this will form into a network of meridians that skirt the scar, and join up with the main meridian downstream of the scar. Whilst this will suffice for everyday living, there will be no excess available and there will always be times when the meridian will not cope with unusual situations. There are organs, whose responsibility it is to see that this happens, and happens well. The Lung pushes Qi around the meridians and is also in charge of the Qi and fluids dispersing out to the skin. If the skin repairs poorly, the Lung has not completed its job properly. The job of the Liver is to allow blood and Qi to flow smoothly. If there is a build up of fats along the blood vessels, or any obstructions causing a lack of flow, then the Liver is not carrying out its functions properly. Whilst it is true that the Heart pumps the blood around the body and the Lungs pump Qi around the body, it is the job of the Liver to make sure that the blood and Qi flow smoothly.

This means that any damage to the body will have to be repaired. The organ to do this is the yin Kidney. If a child falls over and grazes its knee, it will heal well and no scarring will result. On the other hand, if the child is Kidney yin deficient, either through a lack of sleep, or lack of fluid intake, or possibly just a congenital Kidney deficiency, then the scarring will be evident, as the process will not be completed properly.

As we grow older, the yin Kidney begins to be called upon to perform more and more jobs and is unable or unwilling to do such a good job of repair as it did as a child. When you are over

60, the repair function of the Kidney is impaired due to a gross lack of Kidney yin energy. Damage seems to hurt more, repair occurs more slowly and not as well either. The scarring will be larger, and more restrictive of the Qi flow. You may recall that in the chapter on sports injuries, the Chinese system of attending to sports injuries is to shy away from using ice. One of the reasons for this is that the application of ice will slow the repair and therefore retard the Qi flow following the completion of the scarring. Even if the scar is internal in the muscle or tendon, it will be bigger if ice is used to retard the repair. The scar may not be seen from the outside, but it is there nonetheless and helping the Kidney yin to repair will reduce this scarring. If the scar is as small as possible, then the obstruction of Qi flow will be minimized. Importantly, the muscle or tendon will be less likely to re-damage if the Qi flow is less restricted.

Repairing scars is a new practice. From what I have read about the traditional practices, it seems that when a scar has disrupted a meridian, the method of treating the problem is to call on another meridian to take over the job that the normal meridian can't do. However in Sydney, Australia, some eminent acupuncturists have done some good research into scars and found that by throwing Kidney yin and Jing at them, you can flood them with Qi and blood resulting in them becoming much more porous to Qi and the main meridians flow much more freely. How do they achieve this? They needle the scar with acupuncture. By applying an acupuncture needle, a slight damage occurs, and a large amount of Jing and Kidney yin are brought to the site as a consequence of the shape of the needle and the technique of the acupuncturist. This is one of the healing secrets of the acupuncturist, in that the amount of damage is minimal, yet the amount of healing Qi that arrives is far in excess of what would normally be allotted for that amount of damage. In the case of scars, the needle will assist the scar to heal more fully.

As we have seen in other chapters, what happens physically has its equivalent happening emotionally also. Therefore a hurt that you have suffered as a child will not affect you too much but one that you suffer later will have a much more profound effect on you. Furthermore, an incident that hurt you emotionally at a time when you were Kidney yin deficient will have a much more devastating effect than an equivalent event that occurred when your Kidney is strong. Both the damage and the remedy are the same. Whilst the scar cannot be seen, it will still cause the particular organ Qi to flow poorly. There can be Stomach Qi flow problems, that is, a lack of concentration when the event is remembered, or it can be a Spleen Qi flow problem resulting in a lack of memory, or ability to say anything during the time when the old event is foremost in mind. It can be an attack of shyness, when the Lung Qi drops due to an old event being recreated. It can even be a sudden and paralyzing fear, due to the Kidney Qi being suppressed by an old emotional scar.

In a lot of Western psychological paradigms the method of dealing with these emotional scars is to bring them up and expose them again, in the hope that you will be able to deal with them better the second time around. In some cases years are spent trying to find the root cause or the event that created these emotional traumas. Once they are found, they can sometimes get a little better, but they sometimes get worse, as you are experiencing them a second time, and if your Kidney is still weak, or even weaker, the result may not be favourable. There is a good reason for burying some things. Some things should stay buried. But not everything should and this is the benefit of the traditional approach. When it is understood that the way to allow the Qi to flow through and around the scar better is to hit the scar with lots of Kidney yin and Jing, then the answers become clear. This is why sometimes the orthodox approach will work very well.

If the person they are dealing with was young and Kidney deficient at the time they experienced a trauma, bringing it back to them when they see it as an adult, with strong Kidneys is a repairing type scenario. The scar was not able to repair well as a child, as there are always lots of other demands on the Kidneys for children, and was buried so that it could come out later in life and be dealt with when the Kidneys are able to do so. This is what happens, and whilst the individual is still emotionally scarred, they are better able to consciously bypass the scar when they are required to do so by circumstances. Before the treatment they may not have been able to do this, as evidenced by the fact that they sought out a counsellor or psychologist.

On the other hand, dealing with an individual who is already Kidney deficient is dangerous, as these people may simply refuse to find the problem, or if they do, they suffer worse symptoms as a result. These people should be supported with Kidney yin tonics and a Kidney yin diet, so that they are more likely to repair the scar when they find it.

Another method is to simply use another organ to deal with the area in question. For instance, if you are suffering fear and shyness due to a rejection at age twenty, you are unlikely to be in a stronger Kidney yin position at forty, so it is unlikely that you will benefit from this type of "remember and face it" therapy. However a strategy of using a different organ to overcome the shortcomings you are facing is more appropriate. Try to practice using your Gall Bladder and stick to your decisions better, and you will face situations with courage instead of fearlessness. Or, you may rely on Lung and try facing things with a sense of self worth, in an attempt to overcome the fear. You may have a Stomach type constitution and prefer to use stubbornness to get by. Many people use their Heart to get through situations that they fear, and they employ humour. Whatever way you choose, it will take practice and perseverance, as well as the basic understanding that you will always feel the fear and shyness that the scar is causing, but you must employ other organs to overcome it. Best of luck!

CHAPTER TWENTY-TWO

Causes of Disease

Diseases can arise from external problems or from internal problems. There are five external evils: Cold, Damp, Wind, Heat and Fire.

The seven internal emotions are: Joy, Reminiscence, Grief, Fear, Anger, Shock and Surprise.

External evils, (or environmental energies that are harmful) come into the human energy system and cause diseases. The action of these diseases is from an invasion point of view. For example, if there is a fresh breeze blowing, then your Wei Qi, or defensive energy (immune system), can fight off this mild cold and wind as it attacks you. If it is a strong wind, or if it is a very cold wind, you may not be able to fight it off as well as you normally can. If this is the case, you will suffer from an invasion of cold. When this occurs, it is considered that the cold Qi itself has invaded your Qi system. So not only do you have normal amounts of meridian Qi flowing through the meridians, but your meridians now have meridian Qi and cold Qi flowing and sometimes choking the system that is overstressed and not coping. Sometimes it is able to cope. There is a set of symptoms that accompanies an invasion of the superficial meridian system. Provided that you have adequate energy in the main meridians then the cold will not penetrate deeper. If you are run down, not eating well, or over-indulging in your vices, then the invasion will deepen and a separate set of symptoms will manifest.

If the cold Qi is not stopped, another set of symptoms will come up as it enters the deeper meridians. If it is very strong, it will enter the organ's Qi system and make the organ's own Qi excessive and tainted. There will of course be a separate set of symptoms manifesting in this case.

The human system is not as defenceless as this may have made it sound. Every night, the Wei Qi (defence Qi or part of your immune system in TCM) leaves the skin and travels deep inside to remove any external pathogens that may have lodged there. The Wei Qi dredges all of the meridians from the superficial to the deep, and also cleans the organs themselves. This occurs every night, regardless of whether there is a disease or not.

From this you can see that a good sleep is essential every night. Small amounts of external energy infest the external channels every day, with little effect. By sleeping at night, these small problems are removed and do not travel deeper and become bigger problems. Also, most people are aware that if they begin to manifest symptoms of a cold or flu, that a good sleep, or even an extended sleep will have the effect of removing the problem.

Any of the external evils can enter and cause diseases by themselves, or in groups of two or three. You can have a cold wind, or a cold damp, or even a damp cold wind invade. Each will have its own set of symptoms at each level of invasion.

The other genesis of disease is from the seven emotions. These are the emotions that are generated internally by the organ systems and have become associated with the correct functioning of those organs. When these organs produce an emotion, it is at a cost to their Qi. In other words, if an emotion is appropriate, then the organ is willing to expend some of its energy to make that emotion happen. But if that emotion is indulged and becomes inappropriate, the organ will suffer from having its energy depleted. This can lead to an organ dysfunction. In and of itself, it is not a big problem but a weakened organ will not be able to rectify the problem as well as it should. In other words, the control of that emotion is damaged and it is difficult to turn it off. It can therefore persist and further weaken the organ. When it becomes excessively deficient, the organ will begin to demand Qi from the organs that it neighbours. Patterns of deficiency spring up and each pattern has its own symptomatic manifestation.

Let's look at the emotion of grief, as an example. If the person is struck down with a loss, they will grieve. This is good and proper. But if they do not allow this to pass, they will never recover and this also damages the associated organ. As it is the Lung in this case, the Lung's function of self-confidence will be severely hampered and the person's self-esteem will be under question until the matter of the grief is settled. If this goes on long enough, the Spleen will come under fire as well, as the Lung looks around for a place from which to steal energy. Then the clear thinking will go and memory will begin to obsess about the original grief, thus creating a continuing cycle.

The same thing happens for fear, joy etc.

External pathogens are the main causes of excess diseases, and inappropriate emotions are the main cause of organ deficiency diseases.

CHAPTER TWENTY-THREE

Relationships

Why do you like some people, and not others? Why is it that you and your friends differ so much, yet still remain firm friends? What is love, and why can people fall in and out of love?

Emotions are part of the physical body. They do not belong in the realm of the spirit, or the divine. Emotions are closely linked to the body. Feelings and emotions need to be fed just as much as the Stomach and gut need food. In days of old, when people were evolving, it was a biological requirement that if food was scarce, the people became single minded, stubborn and were better able to track, hunt and procure food. If they were secure and well fed, clothed and safe from predators, they could satisfy other forms of emotional exercise, like inventing things, or reproducing etc. Most advances in knowledge have come about when people were safe and living in areas or times that were civilized and secure, and could spend their time and energy on non-essential thinking and emotional responses. This is in contrast to much of our Western "technology" which has developed mainly in times of war, or the threat of war.

If emotions then are physical, they will probably follow a similar physiology to the physical. This was set down in China in the "Declaration of Kan", where a series of emotional requirements were to be met by each and every succeeding Emperor. It was a type of aptitude test for leading China and was all but forgotten over fifteen hundred years ago.

So let us look at how emotions rotate about each other. The Kidneys are responsible for fear. At puberty and sometimes a little after, people are almost fearless and look with disdain at people who have fears or phobias. As they grow older, they become deficient in Kidney energy and begin to make more allowances for things that "might go wrong". With age, when their body does not heal as well as it used to, they fear a lot more things and actions, because they cannot cope with as much trauma, physically or emotionally. Old people and young people do not think the same way and should not be expected to.

When a person is faced with a dangerous situation, they cope with it using their Kidneys, that is, fearlessly. If their Kidneys are low in energy (low in Jing), then they rely on another organ to deal with the danger. They will be scared.

The next organ in sequence is the Liver. When a situation is upon you and your Kidneys cannot deal with it, that is, you are scared, the Liver is asked to deal with the situation. The Liver is the organ of protection and it will protect you by producing an emotion. If the Liver is too yin, or deficient in yang, it will help you to be very placid and you will accept the psychological or emotional trauma and deal with it with depression. If, however, the Liver is deficient in yin or has an excess of yang, the resulting emotion will be anger and irritability.

Remember that the Liver, being the next in sequence after Kidney, is fed the excess energy of the Kidneys. So if the Kidneys are low, then the Liver will probably be poorly fed and also be deficient. In most cases, anger is then a result of fear. For example if your older sister teases you and you fear she may continue to do so, you will become angry with her. If your husband beats you and you fear him, you will become depressed. Also, your Kidneys will become so depleted, that you will fear leaving him as much as staying with him.

The next organ in sequence is the Heart. This organ is King and should control all other organs. Its main function is joy or happiness. If the Liver is too hot and too angry, it will feed the Heart with too much heat, and you will be sleepless and joyless and laugh without mirth. The Liver will continue to feed heat into the Heart, even when it has closed down for sleep and dreams and nightmares will result. If the Heart is fed too little heat, then the person will be cold, unfeeling and exhibit no excitement or emotions at all. They will be pale in the face and joyless. No situation will anger them but none will excite them either.

The Heart is also in control of and is the foundation of self-discipline. All other organs report to the Heart and their qualities can therefore be read from the pulses. So, if a situation arises where the Kidney is fearful and the Liver is angry, the Heart (that is logic, or rational thought, sometimes also referred to as deep thinking) will make a decree, that these organs must control themselves and deal with the situation. So, for example; a child is scared to jump into a swimming pool to learn to swim. The child knows logically all will be well because the adults are there and telling her to do it. Even though she is scared, she must overcome this and do it. So the Heart tells the Kidneys to take some Jing and make itself stronger and therefore more able to control the situation.

Another example might be a tennis player who, during an important match, feels that a line call is incorrect. He fears that if he does not stand up for his imagined "rights", he will suffer more bad calls, so his Liver becomes angry. His Heart knows that this is incorrect behaviour and it also knows that it will not stop any further errors or imagined errors in the line calling. His Heart is not strong enough to control the Liver. He was not given enough lessons in discipline as a child.

The Heart feeds the Spleen/Stomach organs and the Spleen/Stomach organs also feed Heart (which is the reverse of the normal sequence). When the Spleen/Stomach organs are hot, or do not have as much food as they expect to have, they produce excess activity, a lack of sympathy and a stubborn single-mindedness, or intense concentration. Again, a good upbringing will help the Heart to control this selfishness. Often they also produce some ESP phenomena. If these organs become deficient, through excessive eating, or a lack of Kidney energy or a lack of Heart energy, then the emotional response will be an excessive sympathy and a lack of concentration. In its worst form, it will manifest as a person who cares *too* much. Another way to say this is that they become slightly obsessive about what or who they care about. This can manifest in having a propensity to join every cause they encounter, from animal rights, to peace activism, to preserving old buildings etc. Of course there is nothing wrong with being an engaged citizen defending the rights of the underdogs – what we are describing here is a tendency towards a more fundamentalist style of activism borne from obsession and excess sympathy. Spleen deficiency is often associated in the profession with excessive flesh (plumpness) but the opposite extreme can also be true. Many people who run too much, or are on excessive exercise programs, who have trained their bodies not to create flesh, are also in this category.

So, if the Heart feeds the Spleen/Stomach, then self-discipline helps concentration and joy helps digestion. If Stomach/Spleen feed back to Heart, then stubbornness assists self-discipline and fitness, and moderate eating assists the Heart. Finally, appropriate sympathy helps sleeping, but excessive sympathy will only weaken the Heart.

The next organ in sequence, which is fed by the Stomach/Spleen, is the Lung complex. When the Lung is excessive you believe that you are the best. That is, your self-confidence is abundant, you have a massive ego and little things like the truth have no bearing on what you believe. In extreme cases, excessive lung can lead to the ability to be very dishonest, as in used cars salesman stereotype.

On the other hand, if the Lung is weak, then your view of yourself will be poor. You do not believe in your own ability or even your own judgement. Some Lung deficient people have asthma or skin problems and this accentuates their lack of ego. Upbringing of course will moderate both conditions, so that you can survive in society by masking your true feelings about yourself.

The more balanced the Lung energy is, the more forthright and correct living the person will be. If you want to find a place with no crime, go to a place where the people have good strong and well-balanced Lungs. This is why rural people always seem to be, or used to be, more honest. One test of a society is the "Public Toilet" test. If public toilets are clean and fresh, the people are probably mostly good citizens with a healthy sense of self-respect. If they are foul, the citizens are Lung deficient and don't care for the next user, or to generalise, their fellow man.

The Lungs in turn feed the Kidneys. Therefore people with deficient Lungs lack self-confidence and become scared too readily. Their Lungs do not feed Kidneys and phobias develop. To put that in Western terms, phobias are the lack of self-confidence in a person's ability to deal with something that they probably can actually deal with.

Since it is understood that within everyone each emotion feeds another (or fails to) this evokes the logical question; is it possible for one person's emotions to feed another? The answer is yes. If you and two of your friends are talking seriously and solemnly and a fourth person enters the room, with an infectious laugh and a spring in his step, it is hard for you to resist being equally happy. If however, this fourth person is sad, the mood will change and all four people will eventually become a little sad. Therefore, it is quite possible for an emotional energy to cross from one person to another, without even touching. How much more will another person affect you if you kiss, or are intimate with them?

So, if other people's emotional energy affects you, then some energy you will enjoy and others you will reject. Those people who provide you with some of the energy that you are deficient in, you will like to be with. Those people who provide some of the energy you have an excess of, you usually respect, as they are basically like you and make you feel even more like you want to feel.

When your emotions are even and balanced, then a person with a pronounced excess or deficiency trying to drain you, will immediately annoy you. You will dislike these people, but with effort you can re-arrange your emotional energy to allow you to deal with this person. When you are tired or run down, you do not have as much ability to do this and find the person even harder to accept.

Of course, as we have five different major categories of emotional energy, then each of these five levels sends out or asks for energy from the people that you spend time with. Also, as each of these five categories have a yin and a yang function there are a myriad of different personalities and types of relationships possible. It is worth noting that at any given time of your life, your personal imbalances will be different to any other time. For example, to have an excess of Lung yang energy, is not unique but how much is the excess? When Lung yang is sufficient, you are confident, when excessive, you are a little over-confident, but when unbalanced by Lung yin, you are arrogant. If very unbalanced then you are obnoxious and if the yin is really low and the Lung yang really high the heat effects the heart and you are manic. Therefore, to find a person like you, with your type of personality, will be one in 3,628,800. Not only that, but the degree of the organ's excesses and deficiencies will be different. Therefore, it is for all practical purposes impossible to find a personality double.

How about if you look for someone who will exactly complement your deficiencies and excesses? How difficult will this be? It is one of life's mysteries that the enormous statistical probabilities against this occurring are not to be regarded, for many couples do indeed find this type of relationship. In the West, it is called Love. If you find a person like this, marry them; they will be with you all your life. There are two things to consider: (1) If you are in love with someone who complements your deficiencies and excesses, then you will have the same effect on them. I have seen relationships where one person's excesses feed the other's deficiencies but not the other way. This is not love but reliance. (2) If you have any doubts, or feel that you can live without the other person, then it is not love either.

It stands to reason that when two personalities complement each other, then contact between them is beneficial and health giving for both of them. They both become more balanced when together and if they produce babies, the babies will be strong, healthy and balanced.

On the other hand, those people who make love to people not matching or even approximating their perfect complementary personality, are at risk of injuring their personality and even eventually their physical health.

Do not set up house or sleep with someone that you do not like a lot, or at least most of the time.

CHAPTER TWENTY-FOUR

Periods

There are three steps to the monthly period and three organs that are involved. Provided that these organs function properly and are healthy, no problems will arise.

So, for example, in a healthy woman the period should arrive with no prior indication. The bleeding should be clear, bright red and should stop after three or four days. There should be no tiredness or tenderness.

Blood begins to flow down to the uterus and is held in readiness by the Liver, which controls the smooth flow of blood. At a signal from the moon, blood is allowed to flow out and cleanse the uterus. The Spleen is required to build more blood and the Kidney is required to build and repair damage to the uterine lining.

The Liver has the roles of storing blood and making sure that Qi and blood flow smoothly. Provided that the Liver is in good health, then all will be in order. It is the Liver which is responsible for much of a person's psychology. The other two organs are more in the realm of the physical but the Liver is influenced by and has influence on, the psychology of the person to a far greater extent than the others. The Chinese say that the emotions are stored in the blood, so it is not a surprise that the organ which stores and controls the free flow of blood has a large influence on the emotions.

If the Liver is not healthy, then it can cause two general types of problems.

(1) The Liver has a tendency to lose yin, or the cooling part of its nature and becomes hot. This can be caused by (a) excessive stress over a long period, (b) allowing instability and anger to become a normal form of communication, (c) an excessive amount of babies, or (d) an excessive amount of exercise.

If the problem is minor, the blood stored in the Liver will become hot; the bleeding will become heavy and the person irritable, with a dry mouth and red face. In some cases, there may even be a rash on the skin. When the problem becomes more severe, the periods begin to arrive early with slight bleeding. This is due to the fact that the blood is not only hot, but that it has become deficient in volume and is thicker and there is not as much of it. Accompanying symptoms are ringing in the ears, spots before the eyes, sore back and insomnia. If not treated and allowed to degenerate further there will be a gradual decline of the menses. Constipation, dry skin, afternoon fever and weight loss may develop with no lessening of the other symptoms. This person will be fiery, both on the inside and outwardly as they show their emotions.

(2) The second way that the Liver can cause problems with the menses is by not making blood flow smoothly and by not controlling the blood and Qi. The resulting signs are stagnant Qi and congealed blood. If it is severe, there will be distension of the abdomen, cramps which are worse for touch, distended breasts and dark, clotted blood.

If this is not treated, or if it does not heal by itself, then the next stage is to have sudden heavy bleeding or constant bleeding. When clots are passed relief is felt and they will be dark or purple in colour. Depending on the personality and emotional make-up of the person, the progression may develop in another way. Instead of the above, the menses may suddenly stop. There will be distended breasts, sallow face and headache.

The Liver is not the only organ that controls the periods, and if the Spleen is deficient other symptoms will occur. The Spleen has the job of making blood and holding the blood in the vessels. If the Spleen does not perform this task, then blood would ooze out of the veins and arteries at will. Therefore if the Spleen is weak, there will be heavy bleeding producing pale and thin blood. There will be accompanying symptoms of no appetite, watery stools and no spirit (no spirit means a glazed expression, fuzzy thinking and a general lack of enthusiasm).

If this problem progresses, blood and Qi will become deficient and there will be a dull soreness in the abdomen which pressure will relieve. The face will be pale, the individual will be fatigued and the period will produce a small amount of pale blood. If this worsens, the menses will gradually cease and instead there will be a watery white discharge, as well as all of the other symptoms, e.g., very pale face, fatigue etc.

An entirely different way that the Spleen can cause problems is to allow its partner the Stomach to produce too much phlegm. If the phlegm invades the uterus, there will be no period, the lower abdomen will feel full but soft with slight pain and there will be a lot of white discharge. Other symptoms will be nausea, no taste, no appetite and sore, distended breasts. Finally, the Spleen can allow cold and damp to enter. If this is the case, the lower abdomen feels cold and painful. Pressure and heat helps to ease cramps. The blood is dark yet thin and watery with clots.

This is by no means the full extent of the problems that are faced by women. For instance there are over ten different types of vaginal discharge, signifying different types of disease. The main things to remember are that the symptoms of period problems are symptoms of whole body disease. There will be other symptoms which point to the real cause. To stop some symptoms and not address the cause is not sensible. In general, if there are problems with menses then the Spleen, Liver and Kidney are unwell. However, after a hysterectomy, the Spleen, Liver and Kidney are further damaged and it will exacerbate the non-uterine symptoms even further.

To recap and simplify:

The Liver stores the blood before the period and releases it at the correct time. If this does not occur, then the woman will probably have accompanying symptoms like; clots, headaches, constipation and irritability, before the period.

The Spleen holds the blood and makes blood. If the woman loses too much blood, then she will be tired after the period has begun, because the Spleen will be making more new blood and cannot spend the time being enthusiastic about other things.

Finally, there are two types of vaginal discharges to look out for:

1) Yellow and Blood. This means there is toxic heat in the uterus, which may translate into Western terms as gonorrhoea or cancer. You should see a health practitioner immediately.

2) Flecks or different colours with a bad smell. This is also indicative of a serious problem, possibly cancer. You should see a health practitioner immediately.

Refer to diagram overleaf.

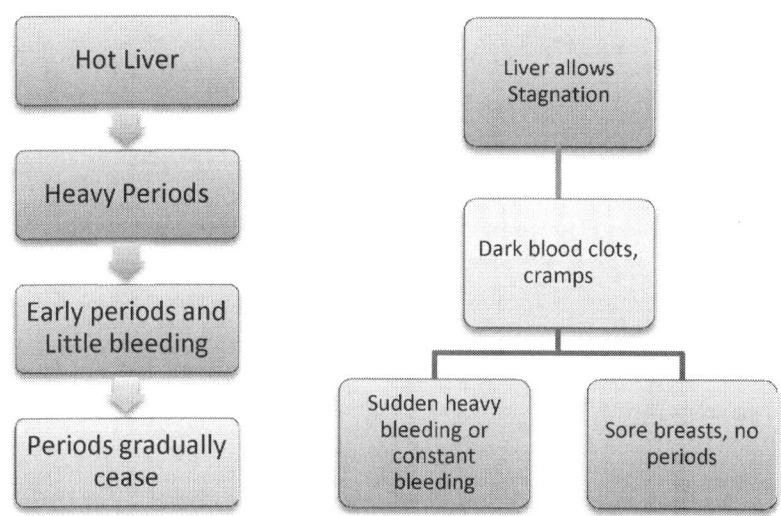

CHAPTER TWENTY-FIVE

Best Food for Adults

Chinese Medicine does not separate the mental or emotional side of health from the physical side. It is my understanding that the Church in days gone by was the supreme authority on all matters concerning the mind and did not allow doctors to delve into that area of their patients. Doctors were only allowed to treat and explore physical ailments. For the last hundred years or so, the Church has lost some of its grip on medicine, and pioneers like Freud and Jung have been dabbling in these areas. Currently, we can call on a hundred different psychological models that try to explain the workings of the mind. The interest and advances in mind-body medicine over the last twenty years have been both remarkable, and more importantly, have become reasonably well accepted.

Chinese Medicine did not grow up along the same lines. There was never any need to separate the physical from the emotional, therefore Chinese Medicine understands that they are inseparable. Whilst the emotions and the physical body are related, they are not directly linked. The concept is that the Qi pattern that is made by the ebb and flow of the organ energies has the function of making and repairing the body, mind and spirit. So a pattern that produces a body that looks a certain way, will produce a personality that matches it. From looking at the body, you can (with training) make a good guess at the personality. Also, when an acupuncturist or herbalist diagnoses a patient he will take into account the emotional problems as well as the physical ailments. Any treatment will be directed at the Qi pattern and by altering the Qi pattern the physical and the emotional will both be affected, to varying degrees.

As it is the Qi pattern that the practitioner is interested in, he will apply tools that alter the Qi pattern. This will sometimes be acupuncture, sometimes herbs, sometimes a Qi Gong practice, and sometimes a suggested alteration of diet. A Chinese doctor then, is more interested in what energy a food will affect once it is in the body, rather than what the food is made from. The constituents of food are immaterial if they do not have an effect on the Qi pattern of the patient.

To say that another way, food is more than just the sum of its parts. Some of its chemical constituents will have an effect on the body and mind and these should be taken into consideration, but this method of categorizing food is not the final word on the subject. The traditional categories for food are of two types.

The first is the temperature of the food. That is the way a food reacts with a person's energy and whether it alters it by heating or cooling. The categories are cold, cooling, neutral, warm or hot. This of course has nothing to do with the temperature that the food is eaten at. It is generally assumed in Chinese cuisine that the food is warmed when eaten.

As an example, take herbal teas. Some teas like chamomile or peppermint are cooling and not recommended for wintertime. They are good for people who are wound too tight. They cool the mind and relax the body, by cooling the Qi that circulates about the Liver. But in the dead of winter, when the body is cold and susceptible to cold infections, it is advisable to try some of the warmer teas instead, such as rosehip, or ginger, or an oolong known as rock tea. In all cases the tea is ingested warm or hot, but the properties of the teas may be neutral, cool or cold.

The second traditional way of categorizing food is by flavour. After the Stomach has digested the food and sent it up to the Lungs, it then separates the flavours from the food and passes them to the Spleen. These flavour essences are separated into five qualities of essence and distributed to the appropriate organs. If you have a problem with the Spleen organ, then you are best advised not to combine too many flavours that are different. In other words, the best meal for sick people is one that has only one or two essential flavours. You can use different flavours for the next meal. Keep it simple as lots of different flavours are harder to digest. If the Spleen is unable to cope with the flavours, or if there are too many or too much of one flavour, it will keep the excess flavours itself. This will damage the Spleen and reduce its functioning ability.

Whilst the Spleen is responsible for the distribution of food energy and essence, it is still the Stomach organ that has the main job of receiving food, splitting it into valuable and waste, and then digesting the valuable parts of the food, before sending it to the Spleen. It is the first organ to be used in the processing of food and also the first to be affected by food.

Let's look at the evolution of the human species. When we were cavemen, we needed to shelter ourselves, protect ourselves and feed ourselves. For these reasons, we needed an organ to be in charge of each of these things and all associated and peripheral actions. To protect ourselves we use the Liver; and to think and imagine, so that we can use abstract thoughts to build a shelter, we use our Heart. For food gathering we use our Stomach. This is an interesting organ, in that it has to work better when it is *not* fed. In other words, if we are sitting in our cave and have not eaten for some time, we need to be informed of this. The Stomach will tell us that we are hungry. If we are hungry, we need food, and if we are not hungry, then we do not. This sounds simplistic, but needs stating.

If the Stomach is hungry, then certain things need to be done. For instance, we find our overall metabolic rate increases. In other words, we are more energetic and our reflexes and muscles work better. We find that we are more alert and have more enthusiasm. We are less inclined to think and more inclined to act. Communication becomes easier and we talk to each other in order to form groups and obtain more food. Most importantly we require the Stomach to digest the food that we do procure, even if it is hard to digest.

So we see that it is a strange organ indeed that works much better and more strongly if not fed and obviously works less well when food is obtained. This concept is unique to traditional medical theory.

At this point we should explore the Western understanding of the Stomach organ. The lining of the Stomach produces two types of glands. The first gland makes mucus and lines the inside of the Stomach with this mucus. This is required, as the other gland makes a very strong acid. The Stomach contains HCL, or hydrochloric acid. The acid in your Stomach is extremely strong and can usually digest whatever you eat. It is a strange thing that if you add water to acid in a laboratory (in fact you add the acid to the water, but that is not the point), the acid is only slightly less dilute. The acid is almost as effective even when strongly diluted. Another interesting item to note from the laboratory is that all acid/base reactions occur faster and with more ferocity when hotter. Almost all chemical reactions work better at higher temperatures.

What has this to do with the Stomach you ask? In TCM theory, they do not have the concept of acid, but instead they use the concepts of hot and cold. It works in the following manner; a hot Stomach means more and better acid content. If you are hungry, then you have a hot Stomach. If you are hungry, you will digest food better, communicate better and have more energy and enthusiasm. A cold Stomach means poor quality acid. If you are not hungry you will be quiet in groups, you will digest food poorly and your concentration will wander all over the place. Therefore, when you eat a meal, you are best advised to wait until you are hungry. Don't eat if you don't want to eat. When you eat, you should eat cooked food, at a warm temperature. Not cooked too much, but cooked to warm the food and therefore assist the Stomach to digest. Whilst a little water won't hurt the strength of the acid, a hot tea taken at the same time will assist the digestion from the point of view of temperature, as well as the ability of the tea to cut through any grease or fat in the meal. Green teas are particularly effective in the digestion of food.

Furthermore, we are capable of making the Stomach work better or worse, depending on what we think of the meal. If we see a beautifully cooked meal on the plate and smell a wonderful aroma coming from it, our Stomach will rise in energy and temperature and we will water at the mouth. Our digestion will be better and we will gain more from our meals. You can further enhance the strength of the Stomach by not talking during meals. If the Stomach is the organ of digestion and communication, then chatting during a meal, when the Stomach should be digesting food will take away some of its energy to digest that food.

The final discussion on Stomach is in terms of time. The two hours between 7am and 9am is Stomach time. This means that for these two hours, the Stomach is at its peak in terms of performance. It is at this time, that it is appropriate to eat foods high in nutrition and energy, as you will usually be able to digest them. So foods such as fruit, milk and whole unprocessed grains, should be eaten at this time, provided that you want to eat them and you are hungry. It stands to reason then, that between 7pm to 9pm, you should be wary of eating at all. At this time, the Stomach is at its most vulnerable and if you are forced to eat at this time, you should be eating food that is very easy to digest, such as: over cooked rice, soup that has been cooking for hours, and food without chemicals.

CHAPTER TWENTY-SIX

Sleep and Heart Attacks

In Chinese Medicine, the Heart is the 'House of the Soul'. The soul is considered to be the true you. If, for instance you call yourself Chris, the true Chris is a small piece of heaven that has descended to the physical realm to be in control of the body that you inhabit. The true Chris therefore resides in the energy centre of the Heart.

This is also how we explain some mental dysfunctions. If the orifices are blocked and they do not see or hear or taste correctly, then the Heart is not given the correct information about the outside world and makes incorrect decisions. This we call in the West, schizophrenia, or mania, or some of the other disorientation problems. When the passageways to the orifices are blocked, it is often a phlegm problem. Many diseases of this nature are not problems of the intellect but rather problems of the body.

When the Heart is hot you have a strong connection to the physical. During the day when the sun warms the earth the Heart remains hot. This is why we say that you should not sleep during the day. As day changes to night, the cool of the evening will cool your skin, then cool your blood and finally your Heart.

By evening time, the Heart should be cool enough to allow the soul to leave the body. We call this sleeping. If for some reason the Heart does not cool down during the night, then the soul cannot escape, the heart will continue to think and control the physical during the night. We call this insomnia. There are many ways and reasons why the Heart can retain its heat into the night. Let us take a look at some of them:

1) The most common reason for not sleeping is to be in a position that is fearful. This is an obvious evolutionary advantage in that when you are not in your own cave and you are in unknown territory, you will find it difficult to sleep. In Chinese terms we would say that the Kidney is low and not controlling the fire of the Heart. When this situation occurs, it is generally considered normal that you will also suffer nightmares and night sweating. These are also common symptoms of Kidney deficiency. Some others will be a ringing in the ears and lower back pain.

2) Another obvious problem that can cause the Heart to remain too hot during the night is hunger. When the Stomach is hot and you suffer hunger, your Heart will not cool as it receives its energy from the Stomach and Spleen, and when this is tainted with excess Stomach heat, the Heart will not cool enough for you

to sleep. This also is probably an evolutionary adaptation that over the years proved beneficial.

3) Another way of keeping the Heart hot is to suffer grief. When you lose something and do not believe that you can continue without it you tend to suffer grief. This grief can be for a loved one, or for a lost relationship, or even for a lost opportunity. When you suffer grief your Lung energy is depleted. When the Lung energy is low the Heart energy rises, which generally means that it also becomes hot. Therefore a lack of self-confidence can cause a lack of sleep. If you are grieving for something, you need to build your own confidence to understand that you can survive and remain as viable as you were before you suffered the loss. Re-building your confidence is the key.

4) The most common reason for not sleeping, especially in our Western society, is due to the Liver. Our Liver is the organ that protects us from outside problems. If work or family stresses you, then the job of the Liver is to cope with these stresses. If the Liver also has to cope with unseasonable weather, and inappropriate clothing, and further stresses, then it soon finds itself overworked. When the Liver is overworked it becomes hot. A hot Liver will heat the blood. As the Liver's job is also to store blood, then whatever position the Liver is in will determine the quality of the blood that flows through it and is stored by it. If the blood is hot the Heart will also be hot.

8) The final way of developing insomnia is to heat the blood via the skin in the same way as would happen during the day. For instance, if you have too many blankets on your bed, or you put the electric blanket on, and leave it on, you will heat your skin excessively, and your blood will become hot. This will cause your Heart to heat also. This can also occur in the middle of summer. Even with a sheet over you and no clothes, you may still find it too hot to sleep.

The Heart has a natural method for not getting too hot too often. This is the yin of the Heart. If the natural yin of the Heart is depleted over time due to constant excessive fire or an overall depletion of yin, then this lack of yin will cause various types of Heart problems. The initial problems will probably be insomnia, followed by palpitations or angina.

The second stage of yin deficiency develops into Heart arrhythmias and strong palpitations, together with anxiety attacks.

If no notice is taken of these problems, then the final stage will be Heart attacks or strokes. A Heart attack is not just fire in the Heart but is a lack of yin in the Heart. That is why sometimes to restart a Heart it is acceptable to strike the chest with your fist, which will reduce the excess yang. However, the best method for restarting the Heart is to increase the amount of yin to the Heart. The Western method of CPR is very good and would be even more effective if you could cool the patient and the patient's skin with all available means. You will note that in most cases of Heart attack the patients sweat profusely. This is the normal response of the body to cool down, which will increase the overall yin. The trouble with this is that the sweating, if it continues, will deplete the yin even further. You can assist the victim if you use cooling methods such as fans or cool water. This is also one of the times where ice might even be of some small benefit if used sparingly on the wrists and neck.

If you do not wish to suffer Heart attacks when you grow older you should look at the reasons why you suffer insomnia. If insomnia is no problem to you at all, you will probably not suffer Heart attacks as you age. If you do suffer insomnia, you should attempt to correct whatever the problems are, so that over the years you do not reduce the Heart yin to the point where a Heart attack or stroke is imminent.

CHAPTER TWENTY-SEVEN

Memory

The Western concept of memory is reasonably unclear. On the one hand, we have people telling us that we all have perfect memories and our brains retain all memories of everything that has ever happened to us. It is simply a matter of training ourselves to recall into the conscious mind all that we require. As this is simply a training problem, we have been trained out of total recall by environmental factors and we can retrain ourselves to recall totally if we try hard enough.

On the other hand, we have the Western concept of the brain as a computer, that is, there is only so much information that is able to be stored in it, like a finite hard drive that can be filled to the brim. This requires a leap of faith, or supposition, or guess that the brain is the conscious part of us and that memory is also stored in the brain. This is a proposition that cannot hold up in light of the thousands of cases of out of body experiences and after death experiences. If you don't have a body, then how can you have a functioning brain? And how can you think and remember?

In any case, "memory" in Chinese terms is wrapped up in the discussion of the Spleen and Heart. As we recall from previous chapters, the Spleen's function is to transport and transform food and waste, as well as energy. Additionally, it has control of keeping the organs and blood in place. They stay where they belong by virtue of the Spleen function. If the Spleen is overworked, or deficient in energy, organs will fall or invert. Blood will spill out of the vessels too easily and bleeding will be hard to stop. The overall muscle tone will decrease.

What happens physically will have its corollary in the emotional and mental situation as well. In other words, memories will not be held and you will find it hard to recall things because they are either not held where they should be, or have spilled out never to be recalled again.

Furthermore, the yang partner of the Spleen organ is the Stomach. It is the job of the Stomach to concentrate (among other things). There is no doubt that memory is enhanced if you concentrate on the event or fact, at the time that it occurs. There are many memory systems that use this fact as a means of enhancing the memory. If you use a system that uses the Stomach to install memory facts into a fixed network, then the Spleen will have a better and easier time recalling these facts.

As an extension of the above, think about the following; the Spleen is also involved with the production of new ideas, and written communication. The Stomach communicates, usually by talking, as well as some sign language (known these days as body language). But what it communicates is dependent on the Heart (conscious mind) and the Spleen (new ideas). Those people who write books or articles, or just school assignments will tell you that there are at least three processes involved. There is the original idea, from the imagination, or previous facts known (Spleen). There is the process of forming words and placing these words on paper (Stomach). And finally, the Heart function of making the words make sense, and conforming to traditional writing values (or not, as necessary), and making sure that when read they will faithfully represent the original idea. There are those among us who are expert at this, and those who struggle to make the words fit the idea. All writers eventually develop coping mechanisms that allow them to do one, two or, on some occasions, all three of these steps together. Each writer will use a different system, depending on the relative strengths or weaknesses of their associated organs. Some will use their Spleen and Heart at the same time having a whole paragraph laid out in their mind and then use their Stomach to lay it down on paper, complete and well written. Others will use their Stomach and Spleen together, committing to paper anything that comes into their head. They will write copious notes and then go over it later and turn it into something that is readable (Heart).

As a word of warning, there is a fine line between the recall of a fact and the fabrication of a new idea. The same organ is involved (Spleen), and it is very hard for the Heart sometimes to differentiate between what is recalling fact and what is being made up. History is therefore open to debate. The history of last week is different between two people. Two people who witnessed an event will remember it differently. What they don't remember, they will make up, and with all best intentions, they will recall the same event differently. Another example is hypnotic regression. Are people really recalling exactly what happened, or are they fabricating some of it, without knowing? The amount of factual recall will vary according to the relative strengths of the Stomach, Spleen and Heart.

Therefore, if you are at school, or university, or simply in a position that requires a better recall of the facts, then you need a strong well-trained Spleen function. It has not escaped the attention of those involved with education over the last two centuries, that those people who do sport and are fit and healthy in their bodies are better scholars (as an overall group) than those who are physically lazy.

CHAPTER TWENTY-EIGHT

Stress

Under normal circumstances, the body functions along the following lines:

Kidney yang energy is used to heat the Stomach, so that the soup (food) in the Stomach is digested and separated into its pure and impure parts. The impure is sent downwards into the rest of the gut, and the pure is skimmed off and sent to the Spleen.

Spleen energy does two things. It separates the flavours, and sends the appropriate flavour to the corresponding organ. It then keeps the sweet flavour for itself. If there is an excess of one flavour, it will by necessity absorb the excess itself. This is why unbalanced eating can damage the Spleen.

The Spleen's second job is to send the unflavoured food energy gained from the Stomach up to the Lungs. This energy is useless until processed by the Lungs.

The Lungs obtain air energy by allowing the Kidney to breathe in. The air energy is mixed with the food energy sent up by the Spleen and turned into body energy, or meridian Qi. The Lung spreads and pushes this energy; much like the Heart does to the blood. Any excess energy is sent to the Kidneys, to replenish what was used in the first place and then any excess is used for forming protective energy. Finally any excess on top of that is used to provide sexual energy. If this is not used up, then the excess is stored in the yin Kidney.

But sometimes things don't go according to plan. If you look at the above process as it is written above, you will see that it is a static system. This of course is a fallacy. Nothing is static. If, let's say, the Stomach is asked to supply energy for digesting a meal, whilst at the same time we ask it to deal with a large milk shake, in addition to supplying the energy needed to concentrate on a written exam of two hours in length. You will find very few people have a Stomach good enough to do this and most will have trouble. What happens is that the Liver temporarily aids the Stomach in its job, by supplying some of the heat and energy needed. Provided that the Liver does not need all of its energy at the time and can spare some, no harm is done in the short term.

Also, there are times in the day when the Kidneys need a holiday, they need to shut down some of their functions. One of these unnecessary functions is the supply of energy for the digestion of food. So if the Stomach is fed food when the Kidneys are not expecting to be asked for extra energy for digestion, it may need to take some Liver energy instead of Kidney energy.

If the weather turns bad and the Lungs need to place extra protection onto the skin, they will call for the Kidneys to make extra protective energy, since the Kidneys may not be able to do this as well as supply the Stomach with its usual amounts of energy. Again the Liver will be called upon to fill the void.

In all of the above cases, when Liver energy is called upon to supply a shortfall, the experience we are having is usually labelled "stress" – in the West.

Stress therefore, in Chinese terms is simply the overloading of the natural system and the application of an alternative power source. This is natural and positive and happens all of the time, at least once per day, every day, for most people. The problem is, that the energy that is received from the Liver is tainted. It is not the proper energy and is artificial, so to speak. There are consequences for overusing this energy; in a similar way to adding caster sugar to a cake recipe instead of normal white sugar. It is similar, but doesn't come out quite the same way.

Also, when the Liver is supplying the other organs with energy, it can't take care of its own domain and eventually Liver signs start to appear. In their mild form they show up as mild frustration, insomnia, anger and irritability. These get worse, until they either get stronger, or become physical, such as RSI, pulled tendons and ligaments, sore shoulders and neck, rashes, purple patches of skin, and lumps and bumps. When the Liver is really overreaching its limits, the Gall Bladder is asked to supply some energy and violence is never far away.

Furthermore, over a long period of time, this tainted energy damages the organs that it is supplying. For example, Kidney supplying the Stomach equals good digestion and strong concentration. But Liver supplying the Stomach equals moderate digestion and becoming overweight, as well as moderate concentration and Stomach ulcers.

When the Lungs are supplied by the Stomach, they supply good energy and a lively body but when supplied by the Liver they promote questionable self-confidence (delusion) and cancer.

This is why cancer is sometimes referred to by Chinese Medicine practitioners as Liver attacking the Lung.

There are those people who enjoy the feeling of stress and can't live without it. They are usually yang people and after some years of living normally they become yang deficient, due to overuse of the natural system. They then find that the only way that they can keep their personality from becoming too yang deficient, is to expose themselves to stress and have the Liver yang fire compensate for the lack of normal fire from the Kidneys.

CHAPTER TWENTY-NINE

Ageing

Ageing is all about the Kidneys. When you are young and growing up, the Kidneys are spending a lot of their energy building your body and repairing any accidents or diseases. At puberty, you are finished making the body and become strong and full of Kidney energy. You are therefore fearless and feel capable of almost anything.

As you get older, the Kidney is needed to cope with the everyday stresses of life and to make a family for yourself. This time in your life is when you need to develop coping mechanisms for the rigours of life and some of these are more damaging than others. Drinking alcohol for instance, whilst it has the effect of dulling the mind and allowing your conscious mind to escape for a while, calls on the Kidney energy to repair a lot of the damage that the poison creates. Some choose gambling, some sex, some worthy causes, some just become workaholics. Whatever the coping mechanism, it will usually be allowing you to cope, but at the cost of your Kidney energy. As the Kidney energy decreases, so does your youth. After a while, you become less brave, as the Kidney is less able to cope with the repair of some imagined physical damage. That is to say, the bruises stay longer and hurt more. When you cut yourself, the scar is bigger, more unsightly and never goes away like some of the scars from your youth may have. This applies physically *and* emotionally.

Once you head towards retirement age, the Kidney is at a low ebb. Enthusiasm wanes, as the Kidneys are not feeding as much energy into the Spleen and you don't cope as change as well as you used to. 'Status Quo' used to be a great band and now it is a great lifestyle!

You are tired a lot and can use a "nana-nap" if you are not at work. Lying down and sleeping, even just for a 20 minute snooze can build Kidney energy, which will assist you for the rest of the day. If the nap is taken at what is called "Baby Yin Time" (between 11:00am to 1:00pm, it will also assist you to fall asleep that night.

As old age approaches, the Kidneys show their lack of energy in much more overt ways. The skin does not repair overnight, and starts looking aged. It gets thin and easily broken. You find yourself constantly worrying about the grand-kids, as there is a perceived threat to their lives on every corner and they are so vulnerable. As are you! The muscles are not repairing as well, and they are soft and not as strong as some years ago. They work more slowly and are much more easily damaged. The teeth are frequently sore and are much more vulnerable to disease. There is the constant threat of the lower back going "out" again and the knees are not what they used to be.

All this is standard for the human race and there are as many variations as there are people. Some people are naturally born more yang than others. They age gracefully and seem to always be younger than their birthday. They retain the glow of youth longer and seem too young to retire when they do. However without the balance of yin, they tend to die younger and usually of a stroke or heart attack. They sleep poorly most nights, and suffer hot diseases, like rashes, headaches and tendon problems (sports injuries).

The yin dominant people are different in that they can carry weight all of their lives, are prone to arthritis (cold in the joints), but usually deal with their lot in life much better. Even though their risk of clogged arteries is higher from less sport and more weight, they tend to live longer and die more slowly. This refers to the balance of Kidney energy and not to the quantity. Those born with less Kidney energy will usually die younger, and those whose parents were healthier when they were conceived will die at a much higher age. That is, if all other things are equal. How much Kidney energy was wasted, or used up during the teenage years? How much was used to deal with a divorce, or the death of a spouse?

These days in the more advanced countries, we usually give older people a raft of Western medicines that are designed to keep them alive. They reduce blood pressure, they thin the blood, they clean fat from the blood, etc. These medicines, whilst often

162

doing what they are prescribed to do, are still poisonous and damaging to the Kidney. The elderly also eat microwaved food, have the occasional drink and are often told what they can and can't do, either by their children, nurses, doctors or nursing home staff, all of which leads to them feeling frustrated by their lack of freedom or ability to look after themselves. This will further reduce the Kidney energy. The Kidney breathes in, and the Lung breathes out. When the Kidney is near to exhaustion, the breathing in will be a problem, and when the Kidney is out of energy, it will not breathe in, and you have breathed your last breath.

CHAPTER THIRTY

Death

In the 1960's, a Swiss born therapist, Elizabeth Kubler-Ross suggested, after many years of observation, that there are five stages of dying for those who are given advanced notice of their upcoming demise. They are: Denial, Anger, Bargaining, Depression and Acceptance. Western psychology and understanding has come to accept these. They are not perfect, and there are many who disagree with them, but they are a good, general guideline.

Some 1,000 years before that, the Chinese were codifying the stages of death in their own terms. This has been done in a few ways, but the most common way to view death is the "Six Division Degradation" method. Just as the meridians, when you are born, open in order and then become strong and influential in a certain order as you grow up, so the meridians deplete and degrade in order too. Rather than the 12 meridians doing this one at a time, the Chinese see them as six pairs of meridians. Each pair have common traits, which is why they are paired, and the best known death cycles are usually described in these terms. The three outer pairs (or yang pairs) are Big Yang, Little Yang, and Bright Yang. The inner three are Big Yin, Little Yin and

Absolute Yin. Instead of the meridians being paired off in their yin/yang pairs; for instance Lung and Large Intestine, they are paired as two yin and two yang meridians, such as the Lung and Spleen, or Large Intestine and Stomach.

So at the end, these pairs seem to deplete and stop in a sequence that is reasonably consistent in most people. Firstly, the Big Yang meridians, Small Intestine and Bladder, degrade to the point of not working at all. Physically the Bladder does not hold the urine, the Small Intestine does not digest food at all and no nutrients are taken from the food. Mentally the signs will be things like an inability to understand ideas and sometimes even an inability to understand another person talking. In extreme cases it may show up as a disregard for facts, which may manifest as a seeming denial of the danger that they are facing?

Secondly, the Bright Yang (Large Intestine and Stomach), will fade, and physically cause a lack of appetite and a lack of holding of the stools. Often in cases of quick death, the corpse will be found in a pool of urine and faeces. Not a nice fact, but often overlooked when discussing death. Emotionally, this stage is characterised by a distinct lack of communication. The person does not wish to talk to anyone or share their thoughts and feelings.

The next stage is the Little Yang meridians. The Gall Bladder and Three Heater meridians close down and cause a lack of fluid metabolism and the body is flooded with large areas of fluid build-up. Emotionally there is no ability to make decisions and the person has to be told what to do, or simply will not do anything. These first three stages may take an extended period to happen, or they may be reasonably quick.

The death cycles then begin the second half and the yin meridians begin to collapse. This half is generally a lot quicker to proceed. The first to go are the Lung and Spleen meridians, collectively called the Big Yin. This leads to difficulty breathing out and muscle weakness. This weakness can be extreme. Emotionally there is a gross lack of self-worth, and an: "I am not worthy of staying alive" type of feeling. This can sometimes be interpreted as an 'Acceptance of the inevitable'.

The next step is the Little Yin meridians, which are the Kidney and Heart meridians. From a Western point of view, these would be the last organs to go, as they are seen as the vital organs and death is defined as the Heart stopping. However, the Chinese see this as the penultimate rather than the ultimate end. Because the Heart energy ceases to circulate, the consciousness fades drastically and understanding goes.

The final layer is that of the Liver and Pericardium organs. This is the Absolute Yin level and the level that holds the Liver spirit or the ghost, as we in the West would call it. The Pericardium and Liver are both protective organs and have protective functions, both in death as well as in life. When any organ's energy is not working, the Liver will supply some of its energy instead, so that the organ can recover. When the Heart and other organs die, it is understandable that the last organs to fade away will be those that are trying to supply energy to the dead or dying organs.

Death in truth is still really a Kidney function. The Kidney in TCM is the organ that takes a person's stored energy and repairs damage. If you are hit by a bus, or shot, then the Kidney energy is drained in microseconds, and death comes quickly. Some diseases take months or years to drain the Kidney, and so death is slow. The Kubler-Ross stages of Anger, Bargaining and Depression are all Liver emotions and will be associated with the Liver organ struggling to keep up with demand from the Kidney's fading energy. This is one reason for the Kubler-Ross detractors, who say that these stages are not always in the same order. They are really all the one stage in Chinese Medicine.

I have one final note on the subject. Those who bravely stay for the end and are present for the final breath, giving comfort and solace are truly to be commended. However, they should be aware that they will need to recover after this. The draining away of the patient's Kidney and Liver will, by its very nature affect the people around them. The helpers will require a special set of Kidney and Liver herbs, or counselling that will offset their unusually drained feelings after witnessing the death. If not attended to, there can be long term effects to those that survive.

Everyone dies. I wish for you all, a non-violent and gentle death surrounded by loved ones.

About the Author

Warwick Poon

DipAc, FAACMA, DipOM, MAc

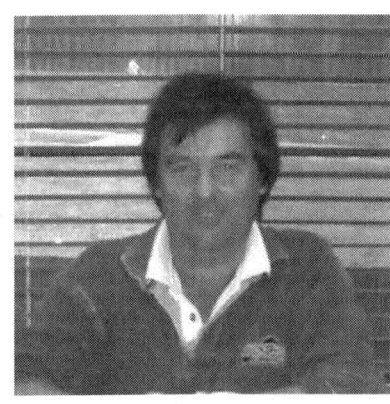

Warwick Poon is a fourth generation Australian whose genes led him to martial arts in his early teens. By the time he was twenty one he had been chosen by his Hapkido master to apprentice in Korean Acupuncture / Acupressure. He later went on to study Traditional Chinese Medicine at the first college in Melbourne to teach Chinese Acupuncture at a degree level and has completed a Masters in Acupuncture at the University of Western Sydney. For the last nine years he has been a keen practitioner of Medical Qigong. Having practiced Chinese Medicine for nearly twenty five years, his knowledge of the human condition and how to balance and manage energies to support a patient's potential is both extensive and interesting.

Contact Warwick at

warwick@understandingyourlife.net

Or visit his website www.understandingyourlife.net

73298367R00103

Made in the USA
Columbia, SC
09 July 2017